DREAMING
OF
ANSWERS

First edition

Published by Brewster Press
Atlanta, Georgia

Paperback ISBN: 979-8-9941451-0-4
Hardcover ISBN: 979-8-9941451-3-5

Library of Congress Control Number: 2026907689

Cover design by Damonza
Interior design by Alan Barnett

Printed in the United States of America

DREAMING OF ANSWERS

UNLOCKING THE
SCIENCE AND SECRETS
OF BETTER SLEEP

WALTER JAMES, MD

MEDICAL DISCLAIMER

This book is intended to provide general information about sleep, sleep science, and sleep disorders. The material presented is for educational purposes only and is designed to help readers better understand how sleep works and how sleep problems are evaluated and treated.

The information in this book is not intended to replace the advice, diagnosis, or treatment of a qualified physician or other licensed health professional. Sleep disorders and related medical conditions vary widely from person to person. Readers should consult their own physician or other appropriate health professional regarding any questions about sleep, medical conditions, symptoms, or treatment options.

The author and publisher have made every effort to ensure that the information in this book is accurate and consistent with current medical knowledge at the time of publication. However, medical research and clinical practice continue to evolve, and new findings may emerge after publication. Neither the author nor the publisher assumes responsibility for errors, omissions, or for any consequences arising from the use or application of the information contained in this book.

Nothing in this book should be interpreted as specific medical advice, diagnosis, or treatment for any individual. Readers should not delay seeking professional medical care because of information contained in this book.

In the clinical stories and examples described throughout the book, identifying details have been altered to protect the privacy of individuals.

CONTENTS

FIGURES AND TABLES

INTRODUCTION

Why This Book?

In 2014, a 29-year-old man with a long history of sleepwalking and a family history of sleepwalking entered the bedroom and then the bed of an unrelated sleeping female at a house party, and had sex with her. She stated that she initially thought that, in the dark, he was someone else; she did not consider this rape until she recognized him after the event. Once confronted, the man made no attempt to flee and seemed to have no recollection of the event when questioned. He was charged with felony rape.

At trial, where I testified as an expert witness, the jury and judge appeared receptive to my attempts to educate them about the science of sleep and sleepwalking. Towards the end of the trial, the jury expressed wishes to find the defendant guilty of a misdemeanor, implying he should have known he might have sleepwalked at this house party—as he had sleepwalked at other times in this setting, and also had a history of "sleep-sex" with his wife many times in the past. The judge denied the jury's request, leaving them no recourse but to find him guilty of felony rape. The judge then sentenced him to life imprisonment without chance of parole. Appeals were unsuccessful.

I have been haunted by the thought of this innocent man languishing in prison for all these years. He remains in prison to this day.

This true story describes the dramatic effects of a sleep disorder that permanently altered the life of this young man (not to mention that of his "victim"). His particular problem was sleepwalking, which you will see later in the book is what we call a *non-REM parasomnia*, a behavioral problem during the phase of sleep we call *non-REM*. I tell this story at the beginning of this book to illustrate that sleep and problems with sleep can have serious consequences. For centuries sleep itself was dismissed more as an absence of internal activity than as any form of active process, but we now know how much more complicated and fascinating sleep is for all living beings, how its perturbation or even minor degrees of its loss can have sometimes devastating effects on the body and the mind.

This book arose from my wish to share with the world the sense of discovery and quiet astonishment I've felt in learning what science has revealed about sleep—a profoundly important, previously misunderstood part of human existence. Our lives involve moving through three totally different phases of consciousness every day... who knew? We think better, feel better, judge better, perform better, learn better, and live better and live *longer* if we sleep better... really?

It was *curiosity* that drove me to devote myself to work in sleep medicine* 30 years ago, and that same curiosity has led me to search out that next new discovery in sleep, that next nugget of knowledge that will move our understanding of the brain and of our life on earth, that may make a difference in the lives of all humanity—because we all sleep, right?

When years later I found that I had one of the more serious sleep disorders, the knowledge gained from all this curiosity seemed like a two-edged sword—on one hand, empowering me to push further in finding possible treatments and cures for myself; on the other, imbuing me with the splash-of-ice-water-to-the-face reality that all the world's knowledge about sleep just didn't happen to include a cure for me... not even one on the medical horizon.

I'm sure that thousands of people share that intellectual curiosity—the delight in learning the next new thing that may affect our lives and behaviors. If you feel that curiosity and want to know what we in medicine know about sleep in this part of the 21st century, this book is for you.

---

* "Sleep medicine" refers to the practice of "internal medicine in the specialty of sleep and its disorders." It does not mean only "sleep medication."

And if you happen to have one of the many common or not-so-common sleep disorders that I discuss here, this book is also for you. Your understanding may expand further; you may find you have new questions to ask your physicians, and new expectations about your care.

In the second half of this book, I explore all but the rarest sleep disorders, and at the end speculate on where these are going, what we might expect, what we might hope for. I do delve into some practice principles and guidelines for treatment in each category and make recommendations for how one might pursue treatment in tougher situations.

You may have chosen this book in hopes of achieving better sleep. Only recently have books on work and life productivity and efficiency begun to recommend better sleep to enhance productivity as well as quality of health and life, and even longevity. The second half of this book contains actionable suggestions for how to develop habits and set conditions for optimizing nightly sleep—as well as recommendations for when to see a sleep physician, and what to expect from him or her for best care.

While this book is written with the lay public in mind, I also considered that many physicians who don't specialize in sleep medicine but want to know more about the topic and its clinical practice (without taking a weekend course somewhere) might find this knowledge fascinating and useful in their practices. Just about everything I, as a patient, would wish my primary care, specialist, or surgical doctor to know about sleep and its problems is covered in these pages.

Lastly, and lamentably, this book is not about pediatric sleep. I believe there is no gift so precious for one's child than giving them a lifetime of good sleep. But the knowledge base of pediatric sleep has exploded in recent years, in parallel to the base for adults, and is a topic for a whole other book. Or books! There are many now. In my practice I usually recommended to parents Richard Ferber's wonderful book *Solve Your Child's Sleep Problems*.[1] It is not new but has stood the test of time and remains a classic. A newer book called *The Happiest Baby on the Block*, by Harvey Karp,[2] suggests calming techniques to help crying babies go to sleep without the "Ferberizing" technique the first book taught, which let babies cry themselves to sleep (and which my wife Monica and I used on both our children, successfully). As a father and as a sleep physician, I heartily endorse enlightened efforts to teach good sleep to our children.

How to Use This Book

If you're here for the science of sleep, if you want to go into fascinating details of all we've learned in the last 75 years (really the last few centuries) about sleep, then you will enjoy starting with the first half of the book, Part One. In it we talk about what sleep is, what its parts are, what it does for us and what happens when we don't get enough. We discuss how sleep is important for memory and learning, for mood, cognition, and emotional stability, and for general health. We delve into what dreams are and how some animals sleep. We connect our sleep with the light/dark cycle of the earth's travel around the sun. And lastly, we try to answer The Big Question: Why do we sleep?

If you're here because you or a loved one struggles with feeling too sleepy or not getting enough sleep, then you can start with Part Two. There we talk about all the major sleep problems humans are prone to—some of which you've probably never heard of—and I make recommendations for how to get the most up-to-date and effective treatment, based on having practiced in sleep medicine for 30 years. If you feel bogged down in some of the discussions of a particular disorder, like insomnia, you may wish to use the Index to refer back to specific explanations in Part One.

Either way, our goal is better sleep—for you, and for everyone.

References for the readers who want more information on selected topics are listed at the end of each chapter as endnotes. A glossary of key terms and abbreviations appears at the end of the book.

Meeting sleep medicine

Not only did I have no interest in "sleep medicine"—I had never heard of it.

And then, sleep medicine and I met, almost by accident. I had trained in pulmonary and critical care medicine in the 1970s, had gone into private practice initially in California and subsequently in my hometown, Atlanta, and was as busy as I could be caring for patients with acute and chronic lung diseases and critical illnesses. In 1991, I went to a week-long meeting of the American College of Chest Physicians, as I and many of my colleagues did each year to keep up with the latest research in our field. Between talks on lung cancer and emphysema and asthma, by chance I wandered into a lecture on sleep medicine, and after listening for a few minutes was struck by the *newness* of "sleep" as an intellectual pursuit.

Where had this come from? After an introduction to the physiology of sleep and some of the medical problems that can arise during sleep, the speaker described sleep apnea, the most common breathing disorder during sleep. This was an obvious link to lung disease (though sleep apnea is not a disease of the lung, *per se*), so it was easy to see why he was speaking at that particular meeting. Pulmonologists were a natural fit for patients with a life-threatening breathing disorder—particularly for one no one had even heard of until recently. That was the moment when my interest in sleep sprouted,* and within a few months I had decided to pursue formal training in sleep medicine. Five years later I was board-certified in sleep medicine, and for the next 26 years took care of patients with sleep problems of all kinds.

---

* Though this was not everyone's reaction. The fellow sitting next to me in the lecture, a pulmonologist from the Mid-west, leaned over near the end of the lecture to whisper to me, "This is junk. Who cares about sleep? Why would anyone want to stay up all night studying sleepers?" Then he left. Clearly sleep medicine was not for everyone.

Those preparatory years, starting in 1991, were not without challenge. In those days the board exams were given in two all-day parts separated by a year, and I knew it would take me a few years to meet the strict qualifications for entrance into the exams. I planned to take Part I in 1995 and Part II in 1996. To qualify I needed to acquire a wealth of knowledge in sleep medicine and I needed hands-on experience, which meant driving across Atlanta every Tuesday for five years to meet at another hospital with a group of physicians who had already passed the boards—to discuss their patients and review their sleep studies with them.

It meant going to as many national meetings of The American Academy of Sleep Medicine in various cities, and local meetings of the Southern Sleep Society in various cities, and as many board exam review courses in Palo Alto as I possibly could. And it meant working with the relevant committees in my hospital in Atlanta to encourage them to see the exciting future of sleep medicine the way I did—to persuade them to let me start a sleep laboratory there.

And during all this time, I was practicing pulmonary and critical care medicine full time, including night call and weekend call. And trying to be a good dad!

It was a busy time. Every day I would come home from work, kiss my wife Monica (and daughter Caroline, born in 1993), and then hole up in my home office with my sleep texts and sleep literature, articles and sleep meeting notes, trying to absorb all the moving parts of sleep medicine. I made hundreds of flashcards to help myself learn all the fields sleep medicine impacted: internal medicine, surgery, neurology, psychiatry, pharmacology, pediatrics, cardiology, urology, otolaryngology, immunology, and my own specialty: pulmonology. Not surprisingly, and ironically, I sometimes fell asleep trying to absorb all I could about sleep.

I reached the home stretch in 1995. Part I of the exam was to be given in October 1995 in Philadelphia, and I had finally qualified to apply for the exam. But then came a revelation: the date of the exam was the same as the date our second child, my son Walt, was due to be born! After a moment of panic, I saw that I had three choices: I could miss Walt's birth (a paternalistic, 1920's approach to fatherhood); I could postpone taking the exam for a year; or I could petition the Board of Sleep Medicine to allow me a later date to take the exam.

None of those seemed the least bit attractive. I was not about to miss my son's birth, and I could not see trying to keep up my studies for what would be another two years if I postponed Parts I and II. The Board was adamant that they were not going to make any special exception for me by giving me a later date for the exam. What to do?

There was no good choice. But then our obstetrician stepped in and said, "No problem! As long as Monica is near enough her due date, we can induce your baby's birth as much as a week earlier than the calculated date."

Which is what we did. Walt was induced—and had a healthy birth—on September 29th. I was there, and there was lots of time left for me to get to the exam on October 5th.

But the adventure was not over! Enter Hurricane Opal. Starting as a Category Four hurricane in the Gulf of Mexico, it had come up into the Florida panhandle just after Walt was born, continued unabated over land, now was predicted to arrive in Atlanta, still a strong storm, on the day of my flight to Philadelphia for the exam. The winds came and grew and blew faster and faster. I was able to talk Delta into moving me onto an earlier flight, which turned out to be lucky as I later found out the one I took was one of the last flights to leave Atlanta before the airport closed due to high winds. The takeoff was pretty bumpy, but the flight smoothed out as we moved north of the storm.

When I arrived in Philadelphia, I called home to make sure everyone was safe, but Monica reported, "Trees and power lines are down all over the city and we have no power in the house. I'm here in the dark with a two-year-old and a newborn and you're not here!"

Okay. Major guilt. Fortunately Monica's mom was there to lend a hand, but still that added up to two ladies and two small children, one less than a week old, in a house with no heat or power or lights or refrigeration, and no husband there to help.

I took the 8-hour exam the next day—it was *hard*—and then flew back to Atlanta that evening. From the air I could see that large parts of the city were still dark. On my way home I stopped at a convenience store near the airport and bought a supply of batteries and flashlights, and the next day I bought a portable generator at Home Depot which provided enough power for a few lights and, most importantly, our refrigerator; after three days without power most of our food was spoiling, and a small dark puddle had formed under the refrigerator from melted food. Power was not restored until five days after the storm passed through.

Ultimately, I found that I *did* pass Part I. Part II, a year later, was in Dallas, and was also an all-day test. No hurricane or other disaster intervened. I finished the test, flew home, and waited. Before the final results came by mail some months later, I tried to imagine failing Part II and having to take both parts all over again (that was the rule). *Not* a pleasant thought.

But I passed.

My hospital in Atlanta agreed to let me start a sleep laboratory and to initiate a Department of Sleep Medicine under the auspices of the Department of Internal Medicine. I was starting to see patients with sleep problems, and my journey in sleep medicine had begun. I was joining a select group of physicians and scientists who had become inspired to learn about sleep.

In this century most of those entering the field of sleep medicine are pulmonologists, with a smaller sample of neurologists, pediatricians, and otolaryngologists (ENTs) following. Earlier, in the last decades of the 20th century, it was psychiatrists and neurologists—and a lot of PhDs in physiology and other specialties—who led the way with groundbreaking sleep research; many still provide the bulk of basic science research. The number of sleep specialists in America has more than quintupled since those days, with a similar rise in the rest of the developed world.

Sleep apnea and other sleep-related breathing disorders are now by far the most common reasons why patients seek help from sleep specialists. But there are lots of other sleep problems to be dealt with—insomnia, restless legs syndrome, narcolepsy, sleepwalking, and on and on—and research volume worldwide is at an all-time high. In one good way, sleep medicine resembles obstetrics, in that patients arrive with an issue (excessive sleepiness in one case, pregnancy in the other) and usually leave happier with a big smile (resolution of sleepiness; a healthy baby). Many sleep disorders have a happy ending… not all, but most. This work can be very gratifying.

The public has responded to this new field with interest and curiosity, and lots of questions. Invariably at cocktail parties, once I am asked my specialty, the next statement is, "Oh, you're just the person I need." or "Boy, does my husband need you!" or "Let me tell you about my sleep." Everyone sleeps (or tries to), and everyone is interested. It's a good time to be in this field, and the depth of knowledge gained in the past 70 years is something of a miracle.

A family affair

My family and I may not be much different from other people, but we have had our share of sleep disorders. It didn't hurt that I was trained in sleep medicine, at least as far as recognizing problems was concerned, and to some extent as far as recommending treatment too. But treating family members (or friends) is on shaky ethical grounds.

All doctors are used to hearing the old saying "Physician, heal thyself." It's considered a truism, but is it really the best advice? Can I, for example, always assume I know as much as my colleagues do about a particular medical problem I happen to have, when it's in their specialty and not mine? If they've spent years studying that particular specialty, of which I have only superficial knowledge? And: If I'm dealing with a problem in my own field of expertise, can I ignore the emotional aspects of my own illness and the ego aspects of my own knowledge base and treat myself without help? The contrary quote we frequently hear is "The doctor who treats himself has a fool for a patient." That is, sometimes, undoubtedly true.

At other times, it's just more convenient and just as effective (not to mention cheaper) to take care of a problem yourself. And what about treating one's own family? The same issues of convenience and cost apply, and the same caveats of insufficient knowledge must be considered. The pressures to treat family members can be significant. We try not to, but inevitably we get involved. It's our job, at least as our families see it.

For example: in the first few years I was practicing sleep medicine, in the 1990s, coinciding with the first few years of my marriage, I became aware of my wife's tendency to be sleepy during the day, every day. She certainly got enough sleep—eight to nine hours a night and 30- to 60-minute naps every afternoon—but still felt sleepy for most of the day. In college, when everyone went out after dinner to a bar on weekends, she would go home… to sleep. When we met, she was living on 2–4 cups of coffee daily, which helped a little.

Was this something I could fix?

We put her in our new sleep laboratory for sleep studies, almost 24 hours' worth, looking for narcolepsy or one of its variants (home studies had not been invented yet). In those now-long-ago days, sleep study information was recorded on large paper tracings, folded into large stacks perhaps 30 inches long, 24 inches wide, 8 inches deep, and weighing about 5 pounds (now all those data are digital, on hard drives, much easier to handle). Remarkably, my colleague who did the study, a woman I admired and respected and who had mentored me in my early training days, reported that the study was subsequently lost. *Lost?* How can such a large mass of paper be lost? But it was, and it was never found, and no explanation was ever given, so no diagnosis was made, and no treatment offered.

In the decades since, I can say that of the 10s of 1,000s of studies our lab performed, both on paper and on computer, none were *ever* lost. Her lost study remains a mystery. But the outcome was that Monica did not receive a diagnosis. After lots of discussions, she announced that she was not excited about expending all the time and effort new studies would require, so—she didn't take part. Her sleepiness persists, really unchanged over the decades since.

What do I think she had (has)? Maybe a variant of one of the disorders of sleepiness, such as narcolepsy, or a variant of idiopathic hypersomnia (more on these later), but we will never be sure.

Adding to that, our daughter Caroline, now 32, has similar sleepiness, similar dependence on caffeine, and a similar reluctance to be studied. Does she also have narcolepsy? Idiopathic hypersomnia? Something else? We will discuss these problems in some detail later; perhaps can place Monica and Caroline somewhere in the spectrum of these "sleepiness" disorders.

Our son Walt appears unaffected by any disorder of daytime sleepiness, which is great for him but doesn't tell us much about Monica and Caroline, as the familial aspects of narcolepsy and idiopathic hypersomnia are not strong; what Caroline may have inherited from Monica's side of the family, Walt apparently did not.

Meanwhile, later in the 1990s, after a few years of Monica's reporting that I snored, I began awakening at night and even during short naps during the day with a sense of my throat closing, followed by gasping. Having already cared for hundreds of patients with obstructive sleep apnea, I had to admit that this was evidence of that common sleep disorder: I have obstructive sleep apnea.

Physician, heal thyself? A home sleep study confirmed mild sleep apnea, and I then went on CPAP (continuous positive airway pressure) for a number of years, and slept better (as did Monica). I now use a nighttime oral appliance for mandibular advancement,* with success. But it's an ongoing problem. We will discuss sleep apnea later in more detail.

The most common sleep disorder in the world (unless one counts voluntary sleep insufficiency) is insomnia. Estimates are that 30 to 40% of all adults have some degree of difficulty getting to sleep or staying asleep at some point. I developed "situational" insomnia during middle age, which I related to anxiety from on-call nights and weekends. Phone

---

* Mandibular advancement means pushing the lower jaw forward with dental devices, which pulls the tongue forward and opens the airway to prevent snoring and sleep apnea. More about this in Chapter Four.

calls in the middle of the night from the hospital floor nurses or from the ICU nurses to me, the on-call pulmonologist, could interrupt sleep in a small way, if the problem was simple and sleep returned quickly after hanging up, or dramatically, if the problem was complicated and involved the possibility of the need to go into the hospital.

If I were to suggest a solution (say, inhalation treatment for a patient having difficulty breathing) and then tried to go back to sleep, I usually found that difficult, as I lay awake waiting for the other shoe to fall, that is, for the nurse to call back to report a poor outcome to our attempts to comfort the patient, making a visit to the hospital mandatory. On many nights no sleep came after the initial call, even when no more calls came. The adrenalin jolt that comes from the initial phone call, the sudden awakening, and the stress of problem-solving, was enough to prevent further sleep.

On-call weekends could be worse for sleep. As a pulmonologist, I might be responsible from Friday evening to Monday morning for 30 to 40 ICU (intensive care unit) patients, many in respiratory failure and on mechanical ventilation, and another 20 to 30 non-ICU hospitalized patients. Rounds each day took 12 to 14 hours, and returns from home back to the hospital were not infrequent during the rest of the day or night.

During the workweek before a scheduled weekend on call, just *thinking* about being on call in a few days would affect my ability to get to sleep. This eventually happened on nights when I was not on call, not worrying about the telephone ringing or having to go back to the hospital. Sleep became difficult as early as Tuesday before an on-call weekend, as the anxiety of the anticipation of upcoming stress prevented the "decoupling" from consciousness that characterizes sleep onset.

When I reached 65, this suddenly improved: I stopped practicing pulmonary medicine and concentrated on sleep disorders alone. Night call and weekend call were reduced to a few emergency calls from the sleep laboratory, perhaps once a month. No more anticipation of sleep disruption on on-call nights causing anxiety that led to insomnia. No more middle-of-the-night trips to the hospital. My sleep improved. The physician healed himself.

Then a new sleep problem emerged, seemingly out of left field. I began having nightmares, perhaps once every two to three months, with the recurrent theme of being attacked. Most commonly the dreamed threat came from an attack from a large dog, but at other times it was a terrifying snake or, less frequently, an unknown human attacker. My consistent response was vigorous kicking or punching at the attacker, and I vividly remember that, in the dream, I could never make contact with the dog/snake/person. I can still feel the frustration of trying so hard to defend myself, with the attacker always just out of reach, my kicks always ending harmlessly in midair.

But, it turns out, my kicks were not really harmless. As I was kicking air in my dreams, while I was asleep I was actually kicking strongly in bed, and on a number of occasions made real contact—with my innocent wife. We have a king-sized bed, so the distance between us sometimes allowed for my kicks to miss her. But not always. Imagine my guilt once I finally awoke and discovered that I had kicked her, had frightened her, had even hurt her. How can one apologize for what one has done while asleep? Fortunately, I have not injured her seriously, but the events have been terrifying for both of us. We can't know what tomorrow (night) will bring. We now sleep with an imaginative grouping of pillows between us.

This is a well-recognized sleep disorder called REM sleep behavior disorder (RBD). As we will see later, REM sleep is a part of sleep wherein most dreams occur, and during which most body movements, like kicking, are normally suppressed. In RBD, for unknown reasons, the suppression fails, and dreamt movements may actually occur. Nightmares involving being attacked are common in this disorder, and self-defense fighting activity emerges during the dreams. The result can be difficult for the sleeper, who can be injured with falls from the bed; and especially for the bedpartner, who may be the recipient of punches and kicks.

Monica has learned to recognize a pattern of my moaning that precedes physical movements—probably a manifestation of the stress of the dream of the attack. In struggling with the snake/dog/human attacker,

I can remember struggling to yell or scream, but nothing comes out… In the dream. In reality, I apparently moan dramatically, and she has learned that her shouting to wake me, which doesn't happen quickly, may abort the nightmare and prevent the kicking (and assuage some of my guilt of possibly harming her).

In addition to all that, more recently, I have begun to display what is called "advanced sleep phase syndrome," a process that accompanies normal older age, as does, for less apparent reasons, a pattern of more disrupted sleep. This happens to most adults over 70. This advanced sleep phase translates into a tendency to feel the need to go to bed earlier, and to awaken earlier, than those in middle age. The disruption is manifest by more brief and some longer awakenings during the night, with overall less efficient and less rewarding sleep.

REM sleep behavior disorder, advanced sleep phase syndrome, and sleep disruption all can improve with melatonin, when properly taken. I have benefited from this.

All of the above—Monica's and Caroline's sleepiness issues, my sleep apnea, situational insomnia, REM sleep behavior disorder, and advanced sleep phase—are described to illustrate not only my and my family's personal experiences with sleep disorders but also to show that these are not uncommon in otherwise "normal" people. They can happen to anyone, so an understanding of sleep and its variants can be helpful for all of us. We will be discussing these and other sleep disorders in more detail later in this book.

NORMAL SLEEP

CHAPTER 1

Some Sleep Basics

We just know

When you've slept well, you don't need anyone to explain to you that you feel refreshed; you just do, and you know that the hours of sleep you just experienced produced that wonderful feeling. When you have slept poorly (or seemingly not at all), you understand implicitly that you have just missed some important experience that should have resulted in a sense of well-being, even if it's a sense you haven't experienced in a long time. Something feels missing.

We instinctively know that a good thing is bestowed upon us when we sleep well (whatever that means!), and that that experience leads to feeling better, feeling "renewed," the following day. Life is better, the world more manageable, the problems of life diminished. Similarly, if we fail to accrue whatever that magical effect is during sleep, we feel worse. Life is worse, our futures dimmed, our world harder to endure.

And this concept applies to all levels of sleep quality, between wonderful and none. We quickly attribute how well or how not-well we feel in the mornings with the perceived quality of our just-finished sleep. Something kept us from getting to bed on time last night? Something kept us from falling asleep after we closed our eyes? Something woke us up in the middle of the night, or kept waking us up all night long? Something woke us early this morning and we could never get back to sleep?

We've all had all of those experiences at some time or other, and when we feel out-of-sorts the next morning and much of the next day, we are not surprised. We know from a lifetime of sleeping (or trying to) that one quality follows the other, that good sleep makes good feelings, and bad sleep, bad ones.

But it stops there. Until the few clues we have now, we have never known how sleep does this, why we need sleep, why missing it makes us suffer, why missing it more makes suffering worse. For centuries, mankind has puzzled over this, trying to explain what sleep is, and why we absolutely need it.

At first, the best explanation for sleep was that it was a form of "death." A sleeping person was considered to be in an intermediate state between wakefulness and death—without being actually dead. In that theory, the main difference between death and the death of sleep was the reversibility of sleep: it was a death one could wake from.

Perhaps this is not hard to understand, given that for thousands of years, other medical problems that looked like death, with its accompanying unconsciousness and lack of responsiveness, were also sometimes reversible. Coma, for example, caused by head injury or infection or illness might look like sleep, and also look like death to the ancient observer, and later recovery from that coma was evidence that death, or at least death-like states, might be reversible. Stroke, fainting, and seizures could also mimic this: partial or complete recovery was possible.

So—couldn't sleep be just another form of reversible death or near-death?

In the middle of the last century, a wealth of new information emerged. The sentinel moment seems to be the discovery of rapid-eye movement (REM) sleep, by researchers in Chicago in 1953 watching infants sleep (and having very fast eye movements then) while recording their brainwaves on an electroencephalogram (EEG). Something measurable, something observable was happening in the brain during sleep, and it wasn't death. (In death, the brain waves on EEG are flat—no activity.)

This was the beginning of the understanding that the brain was in a state that was *not* death, but was not what we thought of as normal consciousness either. It was different from both. It was the beginning of a massive effort to understand sleep and all its implications, its benefits and its problems, and how to make it better.

Once REM sleep was perceived, followed by its sibling non-REM sleep (which is, basically, all sleep that is not REM), the world was enlightened (and astonished) by this concept: throughout our lifetimes, we humans (and many other living things) live in *three, not one, but three normal states of consciousness*: wakefulness, REM sleep, and non-REM sleep.

As we shall see, REM sleep and non-REM sleep are as different from each other as each is from wakefulness. And we now know that a normal human lifespan of 84 years will include approximately 56 years spent awake, but also seven years spent in REM sleep and 21 years spent in non-REM sleep. Something important must be happening if we are normally spending all those years not actually awake.

When William Harvey discovered that blood circulated away from the heart in arteries and back to the heart in veins in 1628, the world felt a tremor of miraculous discovery and understanding, a sense that something previously obscure and unknowable might be conceivable, explainable, understandable, and almost simple. The same sense of the miraculous has accompanied all the thousands of new discoveries in sleep over the past 75 years, which is within a generation of many who are currently active in research and patient care in the new science of sleep medicine today.

One of the earliest American sleep researchers, Allan Hobson,[3] said in 1989:

*More has been learned about sleep in the past 60 years than in the previous 6,000.**

---

* It isn't clear what happened around 4,000 BCE (6,000 years ago) that this refers to. The earliest reference to why we sleep I have seen is in 450 BCE (Alcmeaon of Croton, an early Greek writer and medical theorist, who thought sleep was caused by lack of blood flow to the brain).

And it's now arguable that more has been learned about sleep since Hobson made that statement in 1989 than in all of human history before that.

We now have some partial answers to questions about sleep that have perplexed mankind for centuries: What is sleep? Why do we sleep? Why do we *have to* sleep? What can go wrong with our sleep? How can we make it better? I use the phrase "partial answers" because there is still, and always will be, so much we simply do not know, so much we may yet learn from that next experiment, so much more benefit to be derived.

Nevertheless, it seems likely that this era will be looked back on as the Golden Age of Discovery in the science of sleep, as a sudden emergence from the Dark Ages of the science of sleep into a Renaissance of knowledge. We who are living through these exciting times are all delighted to be in the midst of an explosion of information and discovery!

It is this unbridled enthusiasm that underlies the writing of this book. And it's my goal, with this book, to spread that enthusiasm and understanding to the world, or at least those who enjoy sleep, or wish to, and to those whose curiosity extends to a scientific miracle of our own times.

A "miracle" can be something considered not explicable by our current known scientific laws and therefore ascribed to divine agency; sleep itself has only recently begun to be partly explained by scientific laws, and to me that in itself is a miracle.

The first and perhaps the greatest question to be considered about sleep is this:

Why? Why must we sleep?

Going in circles

The question, "Why do we sleep?" has puzzled man for thousands of years. But it cannot be answered without first asking a related question: "What is sleep?". Only if the "What?" question can be answered can we begin to understand the "Why?" It seems logical to approach the answer to what sleep is by trying to find out what is going on during our sleep—in the body as well as in the brain—and try to draw logical conclusions about what that means for our well-being and our longevity.

This immediately circles back to the "Why". The first reaction to the Why might be: because we need rest, because we get tired, because we get sleepy. But this doesn't help: it only leads to: "Why do we get tired?" and "Why do we need sleep?" Do we get sleepy because we need sleep? (Obviously.) But why do we need it? What does it do for us that wakeful resting does not do? (A lot, it turns out.)

But when we begin to try to understand what sleep is, to break it down into the smallest elements we can, to unpack all the changes in the brain and body that occur in the runup to sleep, during sleep itself (and in its different stages), and after sleep, we find ourselves confronting a panoply of events and happenings which may be beneficial to health. And some that may be harmful to the sleeper (or others), and possibly even fatal. Is sleep always a good thing? What are the chances, in the wild in particular, of waking up dead, compliments of some predator, just because we needed sleep?

At times our sleep philosopher is tempted to throw up her hands and declare that sleep is, on balance, not worth it. Think how much more we all could accomplish in life if we never had to sleep? In an average 84-year lifespan, we would benefit from an extra *28 years* of wakefulness, a lot of time in which to do many things. Clearly the advantages to the individual and to society as a whole would be tremendous if we all had that much more time to contribute.

But our brains would not let us get away with it. The need for sleep seems to increase with longer periods of wakefulness to the point of being irresistible. How often has bedtime arrived and you wish for a few more hours of wakefulness to allow more work or play, but sleepiness demands that you stop? You can fight it, but the sleep drive always, *always* eventually wins. *Sleep always wins.*

Some people (especially those with insomnia) claim never to sleep. But studies in insomnia typically show lots of short sleep periods during episodes of wakefulness. The longest any human has gone without sleep under experimental conditions is 11 days, and the health consequences were (apparently) minimal, after recovered sleep. Many people consider themselves "short-sleepers," and many do sleep less than recommended amounts, but studies suggest that most short sleepers carry around a sleep debt that translates into subtle and not-so-subtle problems. Thomas Edison claimed not to sleep more than four hours a night, and famously said that sleep was "a waste of time." But he kept a cot in his office where he napped daily.

Back to the "Why?" of sleep. There's the concern about predators: we are obviously more vulnerable to attack while we're asleep. Having a tiger waltz into your hut while you're sleeping could lead to a night to remember. Over the centuries, attacks on villages and towns would always start just before dawn, when the victims were most reliably asleep. Primitive humans were most vulnerable to being attacked by animals or fellow humans when they were defenseless, in sleep. (The same applies to the animals themselves, obviously; sleep time is the most dangerous time for them too. We will look at their sleep later.)

So one might conclude that something (or some things) that occur in sleep are so important for physical and/or mental health, and/or for longevity, that these risks are worth taking. If the benefits of sleep were outweighed by the risks of becoming a victim while unconscious, we would, by the rules of evolution, have long since gone extinct. Consequently, there must be significant benefits accruing to all beings who sleep, and our goal In Sleep Science is to find out what these are. We keep in mind the quote from Nathaniel Kleitman, considered the father of sleep research:

> *If sleep does not serve an absolutely vital function, then it is the biggest mistake the evolutionary process ever made.*

We therefore start with what we know about the "What?" Once we have a basic understanding of what sleep is, we can attempt to answer the "Why?"

What is sleep?

Dr. Kleitman wrote a text in 1939, revised in 1963, in which he described sleep as "… a periodic temporary cessation, or interruption, of the waking state, which is the prevalent mode of existence of the healthy human adult."[4] Looking back, he seems to be saying, "Sleep is temporarily not wake."

This is the equivalent of defining night as "a temporary cessation of day, which is the prevalent state of the world." Just as this tells us little about day or night, Kleitman's definition told us little about either sleep or wake. To be fair, we have learned a great deal more about sleep since that time, and what little was known then, Kleitman knew. At least he was no longer conflating sleep with death.

Over the next few decades, particularly after the discovery of REM sleep in 1951,* a universal definition of sleep was derived, based on a measure of brain activity, eye movements, and body muscle tension. Roughly speaking, an organism *appears* to be asleep when there is less brain activity (there is a "less conscious state, with less responsiveness to the environment"); there may be jerky eye movements not present during wake; and there is a significant muscular relaxation (drop-off in muscle tension). A "sleep-specific position" may also be a requirement (like lying down).

In larger beings (as opposed to insects, for example), brain activity can be determined by measuring brain waves with scalp electrodes (a device developed in 1928, the electro-encephalogram, or EEG). Eye movements are measured with electrodes near the eyes (the electro-oculogram, or EOG), and muscle tension with skin electrodes over muscles (the electro-myogram, or EMG). These three "-grams" together give us the information we need to determine wake, REM sleep, and non-REM sleep (with its three important parts), and resulted in our "Bible" of sleep criteria, written

---

* Eugene Aserinsky at the University of Chicago in 1951 connected his eight-year-old son to EEG and eye-movement (EOG) leads and stepped into the next room to monitor him. Noticing that his son demonstrated rapid movements of the eyes on the monitor and thinking him still awake, he returned to find his son asleep. This was the first observation of rapid eye movement (REM) sleep and was subsequently confirmed in infants and published in 1953.

by researchers Rechtschaffen and Kales[5] (the "R&K") in 1968 codifying the criteria for sleep. With minimal modifications, the R&K remains the standard for sleep specialists in "scoring" sleep and wake today.

One might well ask "Why do I need complex wave-generating machines to know if someone is asleep? I can tell by looking!" That might be true, but visual observations alone may lead to the wrong conclusions. Do this thought experiment: You are looking at someone lying quietly in a hospital bed with their eyes closed, and from your distance you are not able to detect quiet breathing or see any body movements. It is possible the person is dead; a longer period of observation would help, but a measure of vital signs (pulse and respiration, and maybe even blood pressure) would be more helpful to detect life. You could try stimulation: if the person moves when you touch them, that's a good sign that they are not dead.

But if they don't respond? Could they still be just asleep? Sleep has its periods of (relative) unresponsiveness to stimulation, but if they are sleeping, vigorous stimulation, such as shouting or shaking, should produce some response. A person in a coma might not respond to any stimulation, nor would a person who is "post-ictal," which means just recovering from a major seizure; nor a person just after severe head trauma, nor a person who has very low blood pressure leading to unconsciousness. We need more data to decide.

If the vital signs are good, but there is prolonged minimal, or no responsiveness to "painful" stimulation, a lot of diagnostic measures may be necessary to tell what the problem is: physical (neurological) exam, brain computed tomography (CT), magnetic resonance imaging (MRI), spinal tap, and likely EEG, to characterize brain activity.

On the other hand, if they wake up quickly and are coherent, they may have just been asleep.

Here is a recent Oxford Dictionary definition of sleep:

[Sleep is a]… condition of body and mind that typically recurs for several hours every night, in which the nervous system is relatively inactive, the eyes closed, the postural muscles relaxed, and consciousness practically suspended.

And here is a Wikipedia definition:

Sleep is a naturally recurring state of mind and body, character-ized by altered consciousness, relatively inhibited sensory activ-ity, reduced muscle activity and inhibition of nearly all voluntary muscles during rapid eye movement sleep, and reduced interactions with surroundings.

And lastly, here is a definition from ChatGPT4, an AI-synthesized definition from many sources:

Sleep is a naturally recurring, reversible state of reduced conscious-ness, sensory activity, and voluntary muscle activity, characterized by distinct brain activity patterns and essential physiological pro-cesses that support physical and mental health.

Notice that all of these definitions use information about the brain and the muscles, as well as a suggestion about relative unresponsiveness. These are about as close as we can get to define a scientific definition, without using any of science's tools.

So sleep can now be strictly defined by EEG plus EOG plus EMG—*brain plus eyes plus muscles.* In fact, I can contend that if you give me all the information I need from brain/eyes/muscles, I can tell you just about everything you need to know about sleep. All "full" sleep studies (studies performed in sleep laboratories or in most research) use these three basic measures; home sleep studies, which are increasingly com-mon now, usually do not, which explains why they are less accurate (but more convenient).

Here is an example of a patient I saw in our sleep practice. We will explain the technical terms later in this chapter, but this illustrates how we approach looking at sleep in the lab using our EEG/EOG/EMG tools:

Marsha, a 20-year-old college student, had a full sleep study in our laboratory because she was excessively sleepy much of the day. As she closed her eyes while awake, her EEG changed from a chaotic pattern seen in wakefulness to a pattern of alpha waves, suggesting relaxation. The point when she entered sleep was marked by widening of these waves, as she entered stage 1 sleep. REM sleep, which was early, was seen when she lost all the muscle tone shown on her EMG lead, and simultaneously she showed sharp eye movements on EOG. Stage 2 sleep was apparent when she began showing EEG waves called K-complexes and spindles. Later, we saw deep sleep when her EEG waves showed tall, slow, wider waves, and muscle tone was restored on EMG. Wake at the end of the study was indicated by a return of the chaotic EEG pattern seen before the study started.

In Marsha's case, a disorder called *narcolepsy* was suspected from her history, and supported in this overnight study by the early onset of REM sleep. We will talk about sleep stages, narcolepsy, and other sleep disorders later. But you can see here that information from the brain, the eyes, and the muscles have taught us much of what we need to know to help Marsha.

Wearable devices, like the smartwatch I wear now, similarly cannot measure EEG, EOG, or EMG, but can give me information about my previous night's sleep, every morning, by attempting to tell the difference between sleep and wake (and sometimes even different sleep stages) by indirect means, still less accurately. Their algorithms vary, as do their accuracies, but it seems unlikely information derived through the skin on the arm or finger could ever be as accurate as that obtained directly from the brain, eyes, and muscles. The EEG/EOG/EMG triumvirate remains our Gold Standard for sleep in clinical situations.

Some studies, especially those in animals and insects—where electrodes might be difficult or impossible to maintain, use surrogates to infer sleep. Instead of EMG to measure muscle relaxation, for example, they might use a "gravity-related posture" as an indication for relaxation; even cockroaches appear to sink lower on their haunches (do cockroaches have haunches?) when they (appear to) sleep.

Altered consciousness with "relatively reduced sensory activity" can be inferred from lessened responsiveness to external stimuli, like reactions to noises or touching whiskers or antennae. Eye movements can sometimes be seen in translucent animals even when EOG leads would not work. This all gets pretty fuzzy, but you can see there is more than one way to skin a cat (sorry). More on nonhuman sleep later.

We tend to think of the brain in awake and sleep mode like an on–off switch: either the brain is on, when we're awake, or it's off, when we're asleep.

In reality it's *much* more complicated than that.

The brain is a plane

Imagine a 747 airliner in full flight at 38,000 feet. All the systems—engines to produce thrust, hydraulics to control flight surfaces, electronics to supply electrical impulses to instruments and hydraulics, navigation systems, heating and cooling systems, waste management systems, and so on—are active in a passenger jet in flight. Some may not be turned on (the landing gear gets a rest during flight) and some may malfunction, hopefully noncritical ones: the entertainment system may have failed, or your tray table mechanism may be broken. But overall, the entire aircraft is alive with hundreds of things happening at once, all in good order. There are even some human brains (the pilot and copilot, not to mention the flight attendants), who control all these systems.

We are awake

The aircraft in flight is analogous to the human body during wakefulness: we have active motor systems (our muscles), sensory systems (taste, touch, smell, hearing, vision), balance systems, communication systems, and so on. We have consciousness and decision-making processes to control all those systems. And sometimes not all our systems are working: we may carry on our daily lives despite a hearing loss, a balance problem, or a muscle injury. But we are awake, meaning enough of our systems are working so that we may continue with a conscious awareness of our surroundings and the ability to interact with our environment. To carry on our daily lives.

We stay in stable flight.

Transition to sleep

Now think of an aircraft in different stages of flight. Start with descent from altitude: some different navigation systems may be needed, the landing gear may be activated, the pressurization of the cabin will be changed. Eventually you will not be able to use your tray table. Then the plane lands and is taxiing toward the gate; some of the systems active in flight are no longer necessary. Motor effort from the engines for thrust is far less required; navigation is much simplified, as are communication systems.

Maintenance mode

Next, the plane parks at the gate; the entertainment system is turned off; navigation is inactive; pressurization is off. This is analogous to the beginnings of sleep: some systems are shutting down (motor movements are less, mental efforts may diminish; senses are less receptive), while many other basic systems (cardiovascular, neurologic, respiratory) continue to be used.

Now picture the plane in between flights, in a hangar overnight, undergoing maintenance to prepare it for flight the next day. Some repair or restoration of services of the plane is taking place during maintenance, and some software in the plane's computers will be upgraded, a digital form of learning. While many of the various flight systems are turned off, the cabin lights and heating and cooling systems remain on, and the basic cleaning processes of the plane occur during this downtime. Other electronic and hydraulic systems may be on and off intermittently for testing and maintenance.

Neural housekeeping

Allow me to tweak this analogy a bit further. Let's say the enlightened management of this airline uses their planes for training as well as passenger flights; in fact, they insist that the same crews manage all the flights on this and all of their planes, and they have the crew review the recordings from the black box from the plane to go over details of each flight when the plane is in the hangar. The plane doubles as a flight simulator when on the ground. The flight crews are proud that they can recreate the experience of previous flights repeatedly, at up to 20 times normal speed, to look for errors and ways to improve flight operations. They even review the recorded conversations from the cockpit during the flights, particularly during stressful events, to understand the implications of pilot emotions in flight management. Lastly, during downtimes in the hangar, the flight engineer reboots the aircraft's computer systems multiple times to delete bad data from the hard drives, to remove accumulated errors from the software.

Similarly, in sleep our brains may be operative (the brain is very active, almost as in a wakeful state, in REM sleep) or very inactive (the brain is toned-down in deep sleep). As we will see, while asleep, the brain is strengthening certain learning pathways and pruning others to optimize memory. Cleansing mechanisms are instituted as they require cellular changes that apparently can occur only while the brain is "offline," not so much during wakefulness. As of the time of this writing (early 2026), we are just now learning about this.

Some brain systems (such as those promoting wakefulness) are not used during sleep or are turned down, but there is never a time when all our systems are entirely off unless the brain is dead. I suppose this is analogous to a plane crash—certainly all systems stop then—but let's not go there. May we all function in the air and rest in the hangar for many years!

To summarize, we can think of the plane in full flight, with all systems on, like wakefulness in humans; transitioning from flight altitude to landing resembles humans transitioning into sleep, with fewer systems needed; parking in the hangar is similar to full sleep, as different and perhaps slightly fewer systems are needed. These stages of flight (full flight, transition to landing, and full stop on the ground) have an (imperfect) parallel with the stages of sleep; as we will see, some aspects (stages) of sleep are more active than others.

All the world's a stage

There's much interest in sleep stages these days. Conversations at cocktail parties about sleep, now a common topic especially as more people have smartwatches that analyze their sleep, frequently come to "How do

I get more REM sleep?" "Am I getting enough deep sleep?" "Isn't REM sleep the most restful?" Everyone seems interested in sleep stages, but few understand them.

Sleep stages (which means distinct *phases* of sleep), as we now understand them, were first delineated* by Bill Dement, along with Drs. Kleitman and Aserinsky, in Chicago in the 1950s. He describes that experience in his delightful memoir from 1992.[6]

Remember how we use the EEG to tell us about the brain in sleep? We do that by putting electrodes (sensors) on the scalp to detect electrical signals from the brain; it turns out the brain puts out electrical impulses *continuously*, 24/7, and these show up on the EEG screen as "waves," which are squiggly up-and-down lines reflecting voltage changes (see **Figure 2**, page 58); the upper four channels are EEG outputs). High voltage means higher waves (taller squiggles), and lower voltage lower ones. The "frequency" of a wave is how often it changes from up to down and back.

We use "histograms" to follow the flow of a patient's sleep during a sleep study. A histogram is a map of sleep "architecture," showing the movements in and out of sleep stages, including wake, during a single sleep period. (See **Figure 1**, page 33.)

Stage W is awake. We refer to this stage as Stage W, Stage Wake, or just Wake. Brain waves in wake are low voltage with lots of different frequencies, with lots of movement artifact (muscle movements cause big swings in electrical signals on the scalp). If we close our eyes when awake, most (but not all of us) show **alpha waves** (a very regular wave) on EEG, which are easy to see. Alpha waves have been used to detect "wakeful relaxation," but many people make alpha waves anytime they close their eyes.

The brain waves from a person who is awake with their eyes open look chaotic, meaning lots of up-and-down in no particular pattern;

---

* Delineated as we now know them. In the Upanishads, Indian philosophical writings from 700–500 BCE, sleep was a state of the soul connecting to universal consciousness. Three states of human consciousness were considered: wake, dreaming, and deep sleep, when the universal consciousness is finally met. I find this astounding, given what we know now about sleep stages.

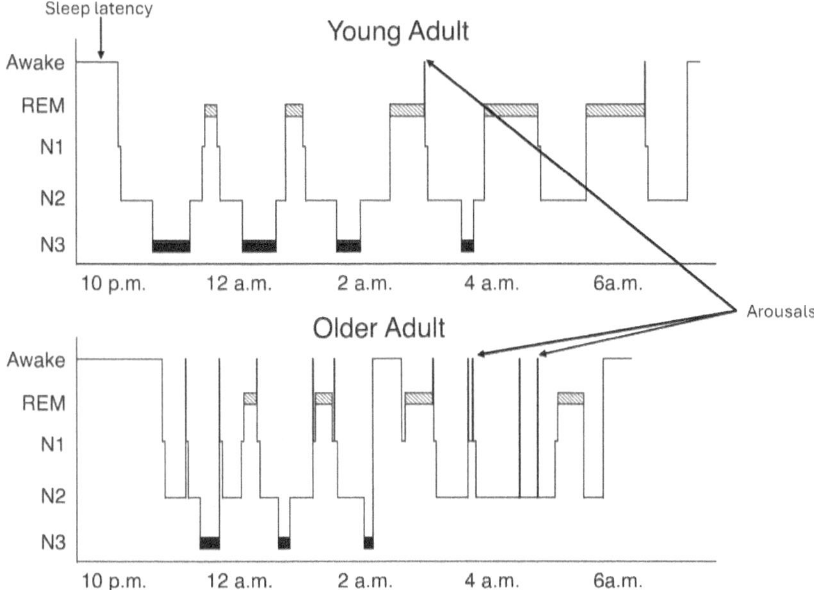

FIGURE 1. Sleep histograms for a normal young adult (age 20-40) and a normal older adult (age 60+). The time of night is on the horizontal axis and the sleep stages on the vertical axis. The length of each horizontal line segment denotes the amount of time spent in that sleep stage. Note that the older adult may take longer to fall asleep (longer "sleep latency," meaning more time spent awake before sleep onset) and may have less REM sleep overall and less N3 sleep, though the recurring patterns of both are similar. Deep sleep occurs mostly in the first half of the night, especially with older age. REM sleep episodes are mostly in the last two-thirds of the night and tend to lengthen with each period. All normal sleepers have a few brief awakenings ("arousals," noted by sharp spikes into wake) out of N2, N3, or REM; older sleepers have more. Overall total sleep time in the older person tends to be less.

this is analogous to an orchestra during warmup before a symphony, with lots of unrelated notes being played and no real harmony apparent. Following this thought, alpha waves with their simple regularity are analogous to that same orchestra now playing the same note (usually an A440 note) following the lead of the concertmaster, slowly over and over, in tuning their instruments. Hearing this is a signal that the orchestra is about to play something truly organized (like a real symphony);

similarly, seeing alpha waves is a signal that the brain is about to move into something more organized, like sleep.

Stage N1 is called "transitional sleep." We almost aways slip through stage N1 sleep on the way into deeper stages, and the first thing we see on EEG as one transitions into deeper stages is the disappearance of alpha waves, and other waves start to slow and weaken (appear smaller). In stage N1, as we close our eyes and begin to fall asleep, we begin a process of lessened involvement with our environment and more muscle relaxation.

> *Alan is sitting up in bed, reading a newspaper, late in the evening. His wife Gloria crosses the room to go into the bathroom. When she emerges, she sees her husband is awake.*
> *She says, "Oh, you're awake."*
> *He responds, "Of course I am. I'm reading the paper."*
> *She: "But you were asleep when I came in. I heard you snoring!"*
> *He: "That's impossible. I heard you walk across the room to the bathroom. I couldn't have been asleep."*

Who's right?

They *both* are. She did hear him snoring when she walked across the room, but she couldn't see his eyes because of the paper. They were closed. He was aware of her walking across the room, as his hearing was still active, and he was able to maintain memory of the sounds. But he had briefly entered transitional sleep so that early muscle relaxation promoted his snoring, which he did not hear, and which he did not remember. He woke when she came out of the bathroom and, having slept so briefly, was not aware he had ever been asleep. So he was right: he was awake (part of the time, partly awake, in transition); and she was right: he was asleep when he was snoring… at least partially.

Transitional sleep is a process of letting go.

Stage N2 is called "shallow sleep" or "light sleep," but it's a misnomer. It's not shallow or light in the sense that it isn't valuable (we spend more time in N2 sleep than any other stage), or restorative (we can feel refreshed after a bout of N2 sleep).

Some people call it "core sleep," since it makes up the bulk of our sleep time each night. We normally spend more than 50% of the night in N2 sleep, so it must be helpful. Symphonically, the analogy is music played "allegretto," or moderately fast.

Stage N3 sleep is called "deep sleep" or "slow-wave sleep." We may spend up to 20% of the night in deep sleep, much more as children (up to 30% by age 3), falling to 20% by adulthood, even less for the elderly (5–10%). The brain waves in N3 are slower than in N1, N2, or REM, so if slow electrical waves really mean less actual brain activity, a "duller" brain, then "deep" seems a good word for this stage. In symphonic terms, this is the "largo," or slow and stately music of the performance.

In fact, as we will see, the brain in some ways is more inactive during deep sleep and the body, the motor system, more active, so we casually refer to N3 as "active body, dead brain." We will see later that important things happen in the brain during N3 sleep, so "dead brain" is a bit of an exaggeration!

This is the opposite of REM (Stage R), where the brain is very active (so 80% of dreams occur in stage R) and the body is inactive (in fact, almost paralyzed), so we say stage R is "dead body, active brain." Most deep sleep occurs in the first third of the night. Three things can clearly increase deep sleep: exercise, sleep deprivation, and alcohol. A few drugs promote more deep sleep too.

Stage N4 was used as a subset of deep sleep, years ago, but was dropped later as unnecessary; it was folded into N3.

I can roughly predict the amount of deep sleep estimated by my smartwatch each morning when I wake, based on how much exercise (whether resistance or aerobic) I had the day before. This is a fairly reliable response. One could also use a smartwatch (or ring) to show that the longer one has been awake before sleep onset (or how little sleep one got the night before), the more likely deep sleep will occur earlier and longer during subsequent sleep.

Alcohol also seems to increase deep sleep, but at the price of diminished REM sleep and more disrupted sleep: REM is pushed into later parts of the night, and is overall less with alcohol. If we want to increase our times in deep sleep each night, daily exercise makes the most sense. The other two methods—sleeping less or drinking more alcohol—are counterproductive.

Deep sleep is also associated with difficulty awakening (from that deep sleep itself): this is not surprising when we think of the diminished brain blood flow of non-REM sleep, with the slowest brain waves in N3 sleep—conceptually, it's like trying to fire up the brain when it's in its most sluggish phase. There were times in my medical practice when, on-call for the night, I received a phone call in the first hour of sleep and had more than usual difficulty waking and grasping the situation at the hospital I needed to help with; I was not surprised to see the next morning that my smartwatch confirmed an awakening out of deep sleep at that time.

More on this later.

Stage R is REM sleep, where we normally spend 20–25% of our sleep (much more in infants: up to 50%). The EEG waves are faster and a bit less organized than in non-REM stages, so our orchestra is now playing "vivace," which is lively and fast.

The differences between REM sleep and non-REM sleep—in both the brain and the body—are quite dramatic. Let's start with cardiovascular differences: in non-REM sleep, blood pressure and heart rate slow, and brain temperature falls (consistent with less activity); a few simple dreams may occur. In REM sleep, blood pressure and heart rate can go up and down ("heart-rate variability" is a key measure), brain blood flow increases, brain temperature rises, and frequent, more complex dreams occur.

The brain in wakefulness runs on a neurotransmitter called norepinephrine (like adrenaline) among many others; norepinephrine plays a role in non-REM sleep too. It's easy to remember how adrenalin "jolts" our system into a stimulated state—think of adrenalin used to jolt the heart during cardiac arrest treatments, adrenalin used in "EpiPens" to jolt the blood pressure up in a severe allergic reaction. But norepinephrine is not there normally in REM sleep, which is under an alternative chemical system, a "non-jolting" system.*

The absence of adrenalin in REM has implications for dreams, as we shall see, and has also been credited for the creativity that is fostered in REM sleep. This switching from two different systems—REM and non-REM, jolting and non-jolting—multiple times a night, are the Yin and Yang of sleep. The presence of adrenalin in REM sleep, where it does not belong, has profound implications for sleep quality. We will discuss the impact of adrenalin on sleep, specifically on post-traumatic stress disorder, later.

The brain is more active in REM than non-REM. In non-REM sleep, especially N3 (deep) sleep, the body is very active, with lots of body movements—arm and leg movements, positional changes, and so on. As we have seen, children have more deep sleep than those in other age groups; if you've ever spent the night in the same bed with a child, you know that they seem to move continuously during sleep.

When a sleeper enters REM sleep, all the voluntary muscles normally become essentially paralyzed, with some important exceptions: there is still muscle tone in the muscles of the eyes (hence the "rapid eye movements"), the diaphragm muscles (but not the intercostals—the breathing muscles between the ribs), and some small muscles in the ears.

We can breathe during REM—using diaphragmatic muscles, (just half our normal breathing motor system), but we can't do much else, muscle-wise. REM occurs about every 90 minutes during normal sleep, but the episodes lengthen during the night, so statistically more REM is bunched up in the second half of the night, and this means that waking up from the last REM period is common.

We will learn how memory of our dreams occurs only if we wake from one, which allows us to describe our dream to our bedpartner (if we've just awakened from one), in Stage R. Otherwise, we have nothing to report.

* This is called the "cholinergic" system.

In some ways, when we are in non-REM sleep, we are mammals, but in REM sleep we become reptiles. In non-REM sleep, we maintain our own "warm-bloodedness," protecting our core body temperature as mammals do, despite changes in the temperature of our environment. Being *homeothermic* means that we "protect" our desired body temperature, using energy to keep it in a narrow range (generally 98 to 99 degrees Fahrenheit, or 36.7 to 37.2 degrees Celsius, lower when asleep) in non-REM sleep, as we do during wakefulness.

But when we transition into REM sleep we are like reptiles, adapting our body temperature to that of the environment, letting our bodies cool in a cooler environment, rise in a warmer one. The body temperature of reptiles conforms with the environment, cold when it's cold outside, warm when it's warm. This is called *poikilothermic*, which simply means "many temperatures."

Now think of being asleep on a winter night under lots of pleasant layers of bedding and a good house heating system. Let's say the home thermostat is set at a comfortable cool setting, but you have one too many blankets on, and your covers are too insulating. Now your body senses that you are getting too warm under the covers. If you are in non-REM sleep, your brain attempts to keep your body temperature at a stable temperature (as mammals do), prompting you, without awakening, to throw off the covers, to sleep cooler.

Now, let's say, some minutes later you transition normally into REM sleep; now you are a reptile—you are now "cold-blooded," and your body temperature will approach that of your surroundings, no longer held to a precise setpoint. Your body cools. That may not be a problem until you and your colder body transition back to non-REM sleep, and transform back to being a warm-blooded mammal.

At this point your brain suddenly, desperately wants to bring your fallen body temperature up to normal, and it initiates emergency measures: shivering. You may wake up completely, shaking violently, maybe even wonder if you're ill—then you bundle up under the covers, try to stop shaking, and go back to sleep. This set of events will occur only with the proper sequence of non-REM sleep in a cool room and too-warm blankets, prompting no covers, then a body temperature drop during REM sleep, followed transition to non-REM, then shivering. This may not be so very common, but it happens. It has happened to me.

The last remarkable difference between sleep stages I will mention here is penile and clitoral erections. Most people are not aware (and might not feel comfortable discussing) that tumescence (increased blood flow, causing erections) is a *normal* event in REM sleep (but not in non-REM) in both males and females. Since we wake from our last REM period many, but not all, mornings, we may wake with an erection, perhaps embarrassingly so. This has been shown to be *unrelated* to erotic dreams or personality variation or any other emotional input.

But it is important to know the abnormal behavior here would be to wake from REM *without* an erection. In fact, in the early years of sleep studies, urologists had sleep technicians measure physical arousal in men in trying to determine the status of erections, which reflected the vascular health of the penis; better testing methods were later developed, so this is no longer done. It is worth repeating that *erections occurring during REM sleep are normal phenomena*, not something to be ashamed of. How many adolescents as well as adults could be spared embarrassment if only this were more widely appreciated!

The way the brain works its way through sleep stages is in large part determined by the timing of sleep. But we relate to our internal clocks in many more ways than this.

Timing is everything

We are creatures of our environment, adapted ("entrained") to the rhythm of the light–dark cycle of our little segment of the Earth rotating in and out of sunlight every 24 hours (or so). Our body and brain are steeped in rhythms.

"Circadian," which means "almost a day," or "almost-24-hours," is just one of the rhythms of our cells. An easy example (and one dearest to our hearts in sleep medicine) is sleep propensity, which is the experience of getting sleepy at the same time every night, about every 24 hours.

There are also *ultradian* rhythms (shorter than 24 hours), like the timing mechanisms of heart cells for a pulse every second, and *infradian* rhythms (longer than 24 hours), like the cycling of cells in the uterine lining flowing into a menstrual period every month. We are steeped in rhythms: we now believe that every organ, and even every cell of the body, shows some evidence of rhythm.

In this book I will try to avoid diving into brain structures too much, but here, in explaining our body's timing systems, I need to introduce one of the most amazing parts of the brain: the suprachiasmatic nucleus, or SCN. These small structures (there are two, like twins, each with only 10,000 neurons; we still refer to them as "the SCN," singular) sit right behind the eyes and are the basic clock controller for the almost-24-hour rhythms of the brain and body.

Light is the single most important regulator of our sleep rhythms. The basic connection between sleep and light works like this: Light coming through the pupil of the eye travels to the retina, in the back of the eye, stimulating certain retinal cells to elicit nerve impulses in the optic nerves, which travel back into the brain. Some of these impulses are to transmit image signals to the back of the brain for vision—that's how we see—but others are sent instead to the SCN, which communicates with the pineal gland, another small structure in the middle of the brain. The pineal gland secretes melatonin, a hormone we casually call "the hormone of darkness."

Light reception and melatonin production are inversely related: light coming through the eye inhibits melatonin secretion, and darkness promotes it. More light: less melatonin. Less light: more melatonin. More melatonin results (in humans) in more sleepiness, but melatonin is not, strictly speaking, an hypnotic: it is not a sleeping pill at normal doses. Instead, melatonin is a *signaling hormone*, telling the brainstem to initiate sleepiness. In other words, melatonin from the pineal gland does not *make* humans sleepy; rather, it signals the brain that it is time for sleep.

In essence melatonin is notifying the brain that it is time to do that thing our species does at night (that is, to sleep), just as it signals to nocturnal animals (like rats) when it promotes nighttime activity (such as ravaging your garbage), not sleep. Basically, melatonin just tells us, "It's getting dark outside. Do that thing you do in the dark."

This is one way that humans retain the circadian rhythm of sleep, by reacting every evening to the onset of dim light, as darkness approaches, to encourage melatonin secretion, and to the appearance of morning light, to stop its production. Each of us has our own individual intrinsic (built-in) circadian rhythm (CR), on average about 10 minutes more than 24 hours, but differing by a few minutes from person to person. Some people have shorter CRs, even less than 23 hours (for example, 23 hours and 54 minutes (which we abbreviate *23:54*), and others longer. This we cannot explain, so we attribute it to biologic variability (a scientist's way of saying "I don't know why, but everybody's different").

Let's say I have that average circadian rhythm of 24:10. I get sleepy and go to bed at 10pm every night. If I get up at the same time each morning and am exposed to bright light then, that light performs the critical role of resetting my inner clock to 24 hours (24:00). That allows me to get sleepy around my usual bedtime of 10pm that evening, rather than drifting 10 minutes later, were I not reset.

In the absence of morning light, my "un-reset" timing (24:10) will "drift" by about 10 minutes each day, so I will get sleepier that much later each evening. If I avoid all light, if I stay in complete darkness for a month. I will miss all the cues that reset my CR, which will revert to its innate span of 24 hours and 10 minutes; my onset of sleepiness each "evening" will appear about 10 minutes *later* every day, and after a month (in the dark!) I will not be getting sleepy until 3am, which is 30 times 10 minutes, or *five hours,* past my usual bedtime.*

For the rest of us, for those of us who are not cave-dwellers, we wake at about the same time every day and then have exposure to light that "entrains" us daily, pushing our CR back to 24 hours, ensuring our sleepy times stay on track.

---

* These results have been proven in experimental conditions (with subjects living and sleeping for extended periods in dark caves, which sounds lovely).

We say that we are daily entrained by light, our most important *zeit-geber* (German for "time-giver"). Other zeitgebers are habitual (such as social) activities and eating, meaning that getting up in the mornings can reset the CR, to keep it from drifting, and meals help with timing too. Both of these are much weaker signals than light.

In keeping with our own CR's—a few minutes plus or minus that of our fellow humans—we each have our own *chronotype,* meaning our unique tendency to be advanced or delayed each 24 hours. "Advanced" refers to "early birds," also known as "morning larks." "Delayed" refers to "night owls." As you might expect, morning larks tend to feel sleepy and go to sleep earlier in the evenings and to wake and get up earlier in the mornings.

Maybe 40% of us are morning larks, myself included. Night owls naturally tend to stay up and go to bed later each night and get up later in the mornings. About 30% of us are night owls. There is also an intermediate ("normal") group (30%) that stays closer to the expected sleep and wake times.

There are measurable values that indicate one's chronotype: one of the most useful is the body's *temperature nadir,* which is the low point of the body temperature's normal variation each day. This normally occurs around 4am daily but will be earlier in morning larks and later in night owls. Questionnaires are an easier way to assess chronotypes than measuring core temperatures.

One's chronotype in itself does not determine total sleep times; it does not change the tendency to need a normal seven to eight hours of sleep per night. But as you can imagine, a particular chronotype could conflict with life's time demands. A common example is night owls, who tend to stay up late at night and then have a tendency to sleep late in the mornings—but if work demands are such that arrival in the workplace and starting work alert and ready to go must happen at 8am daily, their sleep time will be curtailed, with all the subsequent mood and cognitive problems associated with sleep deprivation (more on this later). Late arrivals at work, missed meetings, lack of engagement in meetings and failure to attend to job responsibilities may follow.

People in this group may consciously or unconsciously choose jobs that allow working later or even evening shift work, and do well in it. Night owls tend to like working late in the afternoons or evenings, which may be rewarded in some job cultures. Those with morning lark tendencies are more likely to come to work early and alert, but do not do as well working late in the afternoons and evenings. Some people in management may be less impressed with employees who do not work late. This group does best in day shift work and can be much less effective in evening shift work as their alertness flags in late afternoon and evening.

From a purely circadian rhythm standpoint, almost no one does well in night shift work. We will discuss this in more detail later too.

It has been advised that employers can profit from assessing their employees' chronotypes and adjusting their work expectations, responsibilities, and work hours appropriately.[7] Employees are far more productive and happy when their daytime demands coincide with their chronotypes, when their patterns of alertness and sleepiness coincide with their job and home demands.

The need for sleep is based on timing, and that timing in part determines the pressure our brains sense to look for opportunities for sleep. That pressure factors into the alertness or lack of alertness we feel at any given point in the day, or night.

So much pressure

One way to understand our need for sleep is to consider a hypothetical dial on our foreheads that reads from 0 to 100 which indicates numerically what pressure we are under to quit whatever we are doing at that moment, and to seek a place to go to sleep. A reading of zero would be no sleepiness whatsoever, and a reading of 100 would indicate overwhelming, unavoidable sleepiness, powerful enough to put us to sleep, for example, even while driving on the freeway.

We can assume that most of our lives are spent with our dial numbers, say, in the 80-or-below range, but occasionally circumstances make us more or less alert. We can understand from our previous discussion that the readings of this gauge will reflect pressures from both behavioral and circadian influences.

From a purely behavioral point of view, this sleepiness pressure should increase in a linear fashion from zero when we awake after a good night's sleep to, let's say, 70–80 when our usual bedtime arrives in the evening. We might rarely get into the 90–100 range, as in extreme sleepiness experienced after, say, 48 hours of enforced wakefulness. The behavioral part of the pressure to sleep is dependent entirely on how long it's been since we last slept, how sleep-deprived we are, what medications or chemicals (looking at you, caffeine) we've recently taken.

The circadian part is trickier. There are clock-dependent influences—controlled by our genetic chronotype and our SCN—on sleepiness during the day and night that overlay the behavioral part. For example, there is a normal "circadian dip" in alertness in the early afternoon, usually after lunch (not dependent on food, but food can also play a role); this is also called a "siesta dip," and increases until around 3pm. Then circadian alertness starts improving, peaking at around 6pm, when it starts a slow slide toward bedtime. It continues to drop after bedtime until around 3am, when tendency towards alertness slowly increases again.

We will discuss how we measure sleepiness in a bit, but for now let's just concentrate on our hypothetical gauge. Studies show that sleepiness slowly accumulates during a normal day, so that zero reading at awakening will slowly increase throughout the morning. Let's say our gauge shows a slow increase in pressure to sleep, to a level of 40 after lunch. Now the "siesta dip" in alertness bumps the pressure to 50, prompting a nap (or, less desirably, a cup of coffee).

With a nap, our pressure gauge will show a drop in pressure to sleep (let's say, back to 40), but then begin a gradual increase again to peak at 80 at bedtime. (Interestingly, if we push through bedtime and stay up watching TV or working on the computer, the pressure to sleep in the late evening will *drop* paradoxically (gauge showing around 60) and we will feel less need to go to bed—we get our "second wind."

Eventually, after an hour or so, the pressure will increase again (gauge about 80–90), and we'll finally succumb and go to bed. If we get enough sleep, our gauge may hit zero when we get up in the morning—but if not, we will awake feeling unrefreshed (gauge = 30) and find ourselves wishing to return to bed, even if it isn't feasible.

An important basis of our understanding of sleep "pressure" is sleep researcher Alexander Borbely's[8] *two-process model* of sleep regulation, or drives for sleep, two reasons that our gauge will show higher pressures as the day goes on. The first, called **Process S**, is a homeostatic or behavioral drive: "homeostatic," meaning the brain's self-regulating need to keep itself in a stable, healthy condition, and "behavioral," because we can modify that by changing our behavior.

Basically, this means that how much sleep we have recently had, or how much sleep we have missed, will determine what pressure we feel to sleep, or what number our pressure gauge will show.

The second major drive, called **Process C**, is circadian, meaning that there are noticeable increases in the pressure to sleep based on the time of day, the clock time. There's the bump in the drive that hits after lunch—the need to nap, the sense of a "siesta dip" in alertness—and the drive that hits right at our bedtime, the clock-driven pressure to go to bed at the right time. How often have you felt suddenly tired in the evening, and looking at your watch you see that it's within minutes of your habitual bedtime?

This drive is independent of the behavioral drive, meaning that our pressure gauge will show a bump in pressure to sleep at the appropriate clock times, even if we've recently slept. At any given moment, the amount of pressure we are under to pursue sleep is the interaction of the circadian pressure (depending on the clock time) and the homeostatic pressure (depending on how much time has passed since we last slept).

This interaction can be counterproductive. Consider this scenario, with theoretical pressure gauge (PG) readings: Frank normally gets up at 7am fully refreshed (PG zero) and goes to bed at his usual 11pm (PG 80). Most evenings he spends with his wife reading or watching TV (PG

60 and increasing throughout the evening), but tonight he gives in to temptation and falls asleep in his chair at 7pm for an hour (after which the PG falls to 50). After his nap, his pressure to sleep restarts its gradual increase as he approaches bedtime of 11pm, just not up to his usual peak (PG 70 rather than 80) at this time. He may find that he has an annoying difficulty falling asleep. Once he does, though, he sleeps normally.

The explanation for our circadian drive to sleep, our need to respond to certain clock times, is based on actual "clock genes" as regulated by the SCN, the brain's timekeeper, that we discussed previously. As for the homeostatic drive, the one that varies with how much sleep we have previously had or missed, there are chemical explanations. A number of chemicals produced by the brain promote sleep, and a competing group promote alertness.

Adenosine[9] is a molecule that promotes sleepiness and sleep; adenosine levels increase with increasing brain metabolism and with sleep deprivation.[10] In other words, the more the brain is "exercised," the more energy it uses, the more adenosine is made, the higher the levels of adenosine and the more the drive to sleep. It's no surprise that a prolonged bout of thinking (or studying or concentration) can make one feel tired. The fact that adenosine is produced by brain metabolism would support this: work your brain harder, metabolize more, get tired, sleep, rinse, repeat.

Indulge me now, if you please, for a bit of chemistry class.

Energy in all our cells, brain and body alike, is produced by the breakdown of glucose and other dietary nutrients to ATP, which is adenosine triphosphate, the "main cellular currency of energy" in the body. The "tri-" in "triphosphate" means three phosphate molecules are attached, and we can think of each of those phosphates as a bundle of energy that we can spend whenever we want.

When a phosphate molecule is separated from ATP, energy is released and can be used immediately for the body's needs, such as for muscle contraction, for bladder contraction, for cardiac contraction, even for all brain activity (including thinking). The first and second phosphates each release energy into the region when separated from adenosine, but when the third and last phosphate group is broken off, what is left is adenosine alone, which promotes sleep.* Simplistically, this explains something we knew all along: if we do work, physical or mental or both, it will eventually lead to being sleepy.

Now we see why.

Energy usage by the brain increases brain adenosine, mainly in the alerting centers in the thalamus and cortex, and promotes sleepiness; outside of the brain, energy production in the muscles, as in physical exercise, has been shown to increase brain adenosine in rats,[11] but has not yet been proven in humans. It appears that adenosine also plays a role in exercise-induced fatigue—that feeling that makes us want to stop exercising—a finding that is bolstered by evidence that caffeine promotes longer exercise. (More on caffeine below.)

We can go a step further. Adenosine inhibits brain activity, which means that, functionally, it slows down the brain, as is illustrated by slower brain waves on EEG. Remember those alpha waves we see in many people on their EEG when they close their eyes while awake? Alpha waves are slower than those we see in wakefulness. If the person starts to fall asleep, we see alpha shifting to theta waves, which are slower than alpha; this may mark the onset of sleep (stage N1, then normally progressing to N2, or light sleep).

If the brain waves slow even more, they will become delta waves, which marks the onset of deep sleep (N3, also called delta sleep or slow-wave sleep for that reason). We know that exercise and sleep deprivation cause more slow waves, more deep sleep, and now we can see that this may occur through an increase in adenosine, which slows brain nerve cell activity. That fits: exercise is work; we can spend down our phosphate bank account in exercise until more adenosine is "uncovered," and voila! We get sleepy.

---

* In fact, as ATP loses a phosphate group and becomes ADP (adenosine *diphosphate*, which is adenosine with two phosphate groups), the ratio ATP/ADP falls, which triggers "scavenging" of ADP, "stealing" its phosphate groups from some and giving them to others to make more ATP, restoring energy stores but simultaneously making more adenosine.

The theory that adenosine promotes sleep is supported also by our knowledge of caffeine. Caffeine (in coffee, tea, soft drinks, energy drinks, and even chocolate) is the most consumed psychoactive compound in the world. It appears to cause more alertness mainly by blocking adenosine. It does this by interfering with adenosine where it meets nerve cells at specific receptor sites, not by decreasing or eliminating adenosine in the brain; it fills the receptor sites that adenosine wants to fill, blocking adenosine from causing sleepiness. But this means that adenosine levels are not changed in the presence of caffeine, only sidelined, sitting unchanged in the brain waiting for that annoying caffeine to go away, to free up those desired receptor sites and to let the adenosine do its job on the nerve cells.

Waking up in the morning is associated with low levels of adenosine (a pressure gauge reading near zero), and as that level slowly increases with more of the usage of energy stores that our daily lives require, the pressure to sleep increases, proportional to the "exertional rate" and to the length of time awake. The adenosine level may rise with increased brain fatigue, as the brain metabolizes more of its energy stores[12] in response to hard work and mental concentration, and demands more time to recharge.

If one drinks coffee, the levels of adenosine are still rising but the receptors are blocked; the pressure to sleep is magically lowered—for a while. But when the caffeine wears off and leaves the receptors available for that nearby adenosine, it now makes itself known, promoting a burst of sleepiness.

Some people can fall asleep easily after coffee; others lie awake for hours. This may be explained by genetic and age-related interactions with adenosine; the gene CYP1A2 apparently affects one's ability to break down caffeine. Some of us are slow metabolizers and some rapid metabolizers of caffeine, and our ability to avoid sleepiness by taking in caffeine varies accordingly.

When I was younger I could drink two cups of coffee in the morning, another at noon and one in the late afternoon, and still sleep normally.

Now that I'm older I can drink only half a cup in the morning and none the rest of the day or evening; with any more, I sleep badly. That's the common age-related change in caffeine metabolism showing itself. People with the inherited ability to metabolize caffeine rapidly tolerate a lot of it without problems; slow-metabolizers may take in a smaller amount of coffee but it hangs around in their bloodstream for longer periods of time, possibly interfering with sleep. That's the genetic effect coming into play.

Also related to our daily rhythms are our body temperatures (we have a few). We have already seen that we can use our core temperature to determine our circadian rhythm; we can also manipulate our temperatures with our behavior to improve our sleep quality.

Some like it hot

Have you ever wondered why a hot bath in the evening can make you sleepy? It's not the warming that does it, as it might seem—it's in fact the opposite. The fall in body temperature is what does it.

Body temperatures go hand-in-hand with circadian rhythm; temperatures rise and fall on their own in the timing of our individual rhythms. Sleep researchers speak of *core temperature* (that of the brain and the internal organs) as distinct from the *proximal temperature* (that of the skin of the trunk) and the *distal temperature* (that of the extremities: the arms and legs, hands and feet). When we measure temperature in a clinical setting, either oral or rectal, we are approximating core temperature. That's the temperature that the body tries hardest to protect, since it's the core of our body that is most essential for survival.

The core temperature tends to vary within a roughly two-degree Fahrenheit range (97–99 degrees, even though we think of normal as a precise 98.6 degrees) in the 24-hour day. Important for our understanding of sleep is the circadian influence on this: the core temperature starts to drop in the evenings before or at the time of the onset of sleepiness, and research suggests that the fall in temperature plays an important role in making us sleepy. The core temperature nadir (low point), as we have seen, occurs around 4am each day in normal people and is a marker of the individual circadian rhythm pattern.

Exercise in the late afternoon or evening is associated with an increase in core temperature, and the subsequent cooling that occurs a few hours after exercise has been shown to correlate with sleepiness and with earlier slow-wave sleep. Recall that exercise is one of the most important influences on slow-wave sleep.

But exercising too close to the habitual sleep time makes it harder to fall asleep; this is thought to be because not enough time has passed after exercise to allow the core temperature to fall before attempting to fall asleep. After vigorous resistance exercise, or particularly aerobic exercise, I feel a certain "after-burner effect," a sense of overall warmth and well-being. Sleep during this brief period (1–2 hours after finishing exercise) does not seem likely.

Similarly, a hot bath not too late in the evening may allow post-bath cooling that brings on sleepiness.

During the day, the hands and feet are cooler than the skin of the trunk (usually measured over the abdomen), but the hands and feet normally become warmer in the hours before sleep, with temperatures closer to that of the trunk. This occurs because blood flow is naturally shifting to the extremities as we approach bedtime, as the vasculature of the hands and feet dilates, resulting in warming there. Then, just around the time of lights out, that distal (hands and feet) temperature rises even faster.

Why is this important? Because that difference between the two temperatures, the gradient between the hands/feet and the abdomen, seems to have an outsized effect on sleep onset.

An increasing gradient appears to reflect a shift in blood flow—and therefore a shift in heat—from proximal (abdomen) to distal (extremities), and with cooling of the proximal (abdomen) temperature the core (internal) temperature drops. The higher the gradient—the greater the difference between the skin of the trunk and the skin of the hands and feet—the faster one should be able to fall asleep, as sleep onset is encouraged by falling core temperature.

This naturally leads to the question as to whether warming the extremities can be shown to improve sleep, and the answer appears to be, "Yes." It has long been believed (especially in California, the hot tub capital of the US) that immersion in a hot tub can produce a "hot-tub hangover," a wave of fatigue after leaving the hot bath, leading to better sleep.

Drawing conclusions from this anecdotal information is hard, because the length of the bath, the temperature, and other factors can vary. A controlled Japanese study[13] with over 1,000 older adults compared a hot bath before bedtime, to no bath. (The baths were truly hot: about 105 degrees; the baths averaged only 10–13 minutes.) Time to fall asleep ("sleep latency") was on average six minutes less following a hot bath, which was considered significant.

Other studies have looked at foot baths alone, which also seem to have an effect. What about wearing socks during sleep? A small Korean study[14] (just six young men) confirmed improved sleep with wearing bed socks. These studies suggest that warming before sleep or warming during sleep can both shorten the time it takes to fall asleep, and they illustrate the connection between extremity skin temperatures and sleepiness. Heated foot baths, some with massagers, are now available for online purchase.

Now that we understand sleep rhythms and their effects on body temperature and need for sleep, we should ask ourselves if we really understand what "normal" sleep is.

Normal, normal, normal

What *is* "normal" sleep?

The question of what constitutes "normal sleep" is huge. So much about what is normal, and what is a normal variant, and what is clearly abnormal about sleep is still controversial despite decades of research on hundreds of thousands of presumably normal subjects all over the world. The problem begins with trying to lay down a definition of normal sleep. Let's try this one: "Normal sleep is sleep with the right quality and quantity to allow normal alertness, normal body functioning, and normal mood the following day."

From a researcher's standpoint, this is a mess from the beginning. How do you define "normal alertness"? We will discuss sleep studies later but suffice it to say there are multiple ways of defining "normal alertness," so this is controversial too. Let's assume that this is shorthand to mean not only normal alertness to our surroundings but also normal cognition, normal reasoning, normal vigilance. How do you define normal body functioning? Normal mood? How these are defined may vary from study to study, so comparisons can be difficult.

Here are some other ways normal sleep is defined: "Normal sleep is when you fall asleep quite easily, do not fully wake up during the night, do not wake up too early, and feel refreshed in the morning." This is not too different from our first try. Others define sleep in technical terms: this many minutes of REM, this many of the stages of non-REM, this much overall sleep, this timing within the light-dark cycle, and so on, without mentioning the outcomes.

We can talk about normal sleep stages and overall hours of sleep, but it's important to say at the outset that we don't have a precise way of defining what perfect sleep is, other than subjectively: we know a great night of sleep when we've had one, and we feel good afterwards. In many studies of "normal sleep," the researchers will recruit potential subjects for investigation as those with "no sleep complaint": in other words, those who seem to be doing well during the day, and feel they're sleeping well at night. Then, after testing, they will remove from the pool of subjects any who show obvious sleep disorders, usually including "insufficient sleep" (see below).

We're still seeing that it can be hard to define normal sleep. But let's keep trying. If we consider human reactions to the light-dark cycle, we might start a new definition by requiring that normal sleep occurs *at night.* Is this not reasonable? How could sleep that's not at night be normal when it goes against all our thousands of years of adaptation to the cycles of the sun and the moon, of day and night? But does that mean we can't get normal sleep during the day? If it's light outside but (artificially) dark inside? If our timing of sleep is off for sunrise and sunset but we are careful to keep our bedrooms dark, and feel we're sleeping fine? If we work shifts, and try hard to sleep during the day? Maybe requiring night sleep is too restrictive.

Let's go back to looking at the various parts of sleep, and what we know about them. "Sleep architecture" is the blueprint of the night, the way the building blocks of sleep (the stages) are sized and arranged in order throughout a night of sleep. Normal sleep architecture differs from normal infants to normal adolescents to normal adults, and even to normal seniors.

We can say that most "normal" adults have a few minutes of transitional, or stage N1 sleep, and then enter stage N2, the "light" sleep that dominates the night. The first N2 period may be short, though, if there is a need to go quickly into deep, or N3 sleep. Remember that taking exercise the previous day and sleep deprivation the previous night will push us to go into deep sleep earlier and longer.

After deep sleep, we move back into light, N2, sleep, and then perhaps, 60 to 90 minutes after falling onset we will enter our first REM period, maybe lasting 20 to 30 minutes. Another period of N3 (or more) may occur early on.

The rest of the night will be alternating N2 and REM periods, with REM periods usually progressively longer during the night, until we finally awaken from one of those. We remember only the dreams we awaken from, however, so dreams occurring in earlier REM periods are lost to memory immediately without an awakening. Throughout the night, we may have many short awakenings that never make it into memory—we call these "arousals"—that may result in a sleep stage change, a change of body position, or no obvious effect. We will discuss sleep and memory in more detail later.

Infants may transition quickly into REM sleep at onset and spend up to 50% of their sleep time in REM, whereas adults usually have 25% or less. Children and adolescents, however, spend much more time in deep sleep than adults. Seniors may have little to no deep sleep, and more arousals (and true awakenings). What's not known is whether different, more "healthy" lifestyles (with more lifetime exercise, less alcohol, and better diet, for example, might lead a particular older adult to avoid the deterioration in sleep architecture and the common complaint of seniors: less refreshing sleep.

What about overall sleep time? How much sleep is normal? The traditional answer has been: *enough*. Enough to feel alert and function well the following day (we know how fuzzy that definition is). For adults, the answer now is at least *seven* hours; this comes from a report from a national committee,[15] looking at the world's literature on sleep needs in 2015.

For those of us in sleep medicine who are asked daily to state precisely the proper amount of sleep, this helpfully gave us a number, a minimum sleep time figure we could have our patients aim to meet or exceed. And there is ample research backing up this number. Just as important, it allowed us to define a number that qualifies as sleep deprivation: six hours. I can assure my patients that they are chronically sleep-deprived if they sleep less than six hours a night. Between six and seven? Usually. Above seven? Depends. That may be enough for many people (the committee thought so) but many people require more than seven hours nightly to feel their best.

The committee set out the following guidelines for normal sleep times:

Newborns	14–17 hours
Toddlers	11–14 hours
Preschoolers	10–13 hours
School-age children	9–11 hours
Teenagers	8–10 hours
Young adults	7–9 hours
Adults	7–8 hours

All parents worry whether their children, especially the adolescents, have enough sleep, and there's reason to believe that most, in fact, are sleeping less than they should. That applies to the older age-groups too.

Can we define normal sleep now? Not completely satisfactorily, but perhaps this modification of our first definition above is sufficient: "Normal sleep is sleep with the right quality, quantity, and timing to allow normal alertness, normal body functioning, and normal mood the following day."

To sleep, perchance to be observed

For the person who complains of feeling chronically, abnormally sleepy, sleep studies can be helpful. In this situation, we are asking the question "What, if anything, is going on during this person's sleep period that makes his/her sleep so unrefreshing?" It's a legitimate question, and in-lab and/or home studies frequently provide an answer, and more importantly, can result in treatment that improves the person's quality of life. The choice of study is frequently made on the cost/convenience level, perhaps entirely based on one´s insurance coverage, rather than on scientific enquiry; if a home study fails to show an answer (usually sleep apnea, since that is the main diagnostic strength of a home study), an in-lab study may be the necessary next step.

For those who are suspected of having bad things happen during sleep (like seizures or other abnormal body movements—including sleepwalking) in-lab or home studies may give the answer. Video monitoring, available only in the lab, can be a critical element in making the right diagnosis.

But for those with insomnia, for those who complain of being unable to fall asleep or stay asleep or both, sleep studies are usually a waste of time, effort, and money. If the patient sleeps poorly at home, it is likely they will sleep even less well in a sleep laboratory, in a strange bed in a strange room with wires all over their body and a strange technician watching them all night:

Insomnia patient: "What did you learn from my sleep study in the sleep lab last night, doctor?"
Doctor: "We learned that you don't sleep."
Patient: "That's it? I told you that before we started!"

There is a proviso here, though: if another sleep disorder (such as sleep apnea) is suspected to be present along with insomnia, sleep studies can still be helpful, as that subtle sleep disorder may be contributing to insomnia, rather than the insomnia being "primary." Herein the art of medicine is required to make this decision, by considering the right possibilities, asking the right questions, making the correct examination. More on this later. For the most part, however, for those who have trouble initiating or maintaining sleep, formal sleep studies are not useful.

Sleep is studied in research settings to advance knowledge on what's normal (sleep physiology) and to investigate disorders of sleep (sleep pathology). Furthermore, sleep is commonly studied today in clinical settings to diagnose and characterize what is wrong with the sleep of individuals (sleep medicine). We will get into the problems people have with sleep in much more detail later, but for the discussion of sleep studies, let's lump these into three categories: problems with feeling too sleepy during the day; problems with bad things that happen during sleep; and problems with being unable to fall asleep, or stay asleep.

We can lump sleep studies themselves into three categories: "full" sleep studies performed in a sleep laboratory ("in-lab studies"}, sleep studies performed at home ("home studies"), and everything else. "Everything else" includes your sports watch or smartwatch or smart ring ("wearables") or smart mattress or any other external device ("nearables") that you purchase privately and which purports to tell you details about your sleep.

Full, in-lab studies are the gold standard for examining sleep these days (home studies give less information, though sometimes just enough). The emergence of sleep laboratories in the 1980s in America and across the world signified a sea change in our understanding of sleep and sleep disorders. One of the first "sleep studies" was performed in 1953 at the University of Chicago and consisted only of a few EEG (brain wave) electrodes attached to the scalp of some infants (which is when REM sleep was discovered). The standard "in-lab" study has evolved significantly since then, and now requires a fully-equipped (and fully accredited) sleep laboratory with a central computerized control room and a number of connected "sleep beds," with dedicated, also accredited sleep technicians who spend entire nights observing patients.

A sleep study is also called a "polysomnogram," which just means "many sleep measurements." Remember the EEG/EOG/EMG triad we talked about earlier? These (the brainwaves, eye movements, and muscle tone measurements, respectively) form the basis of the "sleep" part of a sleep study, with each of the data inputs feeding into a channel in the main computer. There may be 8–10 EEG channels, two eye channels, and two EMG channels; in addition, there are commonly channels that monitor breathing by measuring airflow in and out, as well as efforts to breathe, with other channels monitoring oxygen levels and even snoring levels. Heart rhythm is on an EKG (electrocardiogram) channel. There are lots of channels, lots of data for the technician to monitor and adjust all night long, and thus lots of data for the sleep physician to review and interpret later.

In the early decades of sleep medicine, full polysomnographic sleep studies were tried in the home setting (to try to save money, to try to make it more convenient for the sleeper), usually with a technician who would set up the study in the home, and then leave. Not surprisingly, many of these studies failed when the unattended sleeping subject moved during sleep and pulled off the electrodes, with data lost for the rest of the night—so this is not done much these days.

Most home studies now have far fewer channels, and have given up the EEG monitoring altogether. Can you still measure sleep—can you be sure the person is *actually asleep*—without measuring brain waves? The answer is only indirectly, as with changes in heart rate, changes in body movements, and changes in breathing. This is a tradeoff, as the

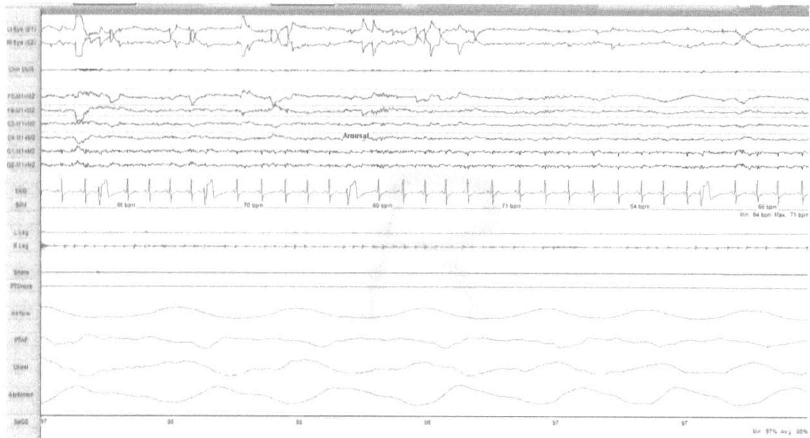

FIGURE 2. A typical page from a polysomnogram in an adult. This page, called an epoch, shows 30 seconds of sleep; there may be over 1000 pages in a study. Each 30-second epoch is scored as wake, N1, N2, N3, or REM, and all the epochs are added together in the scoring process. This epoch was scored R, for REM sleep. The top two channels (note labels on the left) are measures of right and left eye movements (EOG). The third is chin muscle tone (EMG). The next six are brain waves (EEG) from scalp electrodes. After that are an EKG (heart) tracing, right and left leg muscle tone (EMG), followed by two snore monitors, two airflow channels, and two breathing effort channels (chest and abdomen). Last is SpO2, the oxygen saturation measured with an oximeter.

sleep physician can never be sure of the actual, precise sleep time on a home test, but the convenience and lower cost of a home study compared to an in-lab test are thought to outweigh this disadvantage. As a result, home studies now greatly outnumber in-lab studies in most areas. Health insurers figured out early on that these tests cost them less, and now mandate home studies in many situations.

In-lab sleep studies are also useful in finding the right pressures applied to the nose and throat (CPAP pressures) that will reverse obstructive sleep apnea, determining a "prescription" of the right pressures for that individual. We will discuss sleep apnea and CPAP usage in some detail later.

Smart devices or wearable devices, like smartwatches and rings, measure sleep with similarly indirect parameters, and results are still in

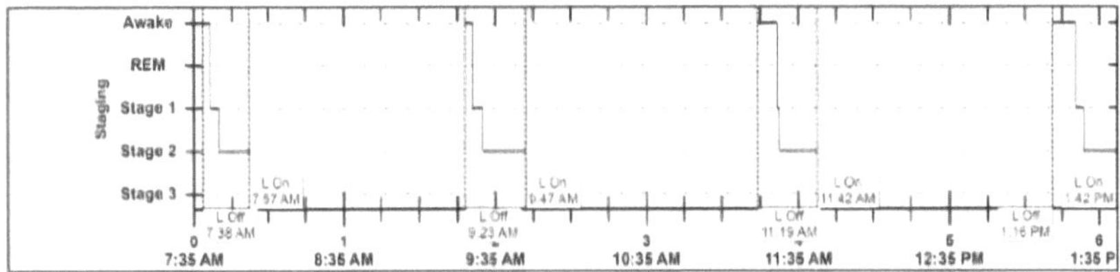

FIGURE 3. A typical multiple sleep latency test (MSLT) histogram. Four naps are shown here in graphic form. The times of "lights off" and "lights on" are noted on the horizontal timeline. The "sleep latency" for each nap is the time it takes to transition from wake ("Awake") to any stage of sleep (in each nap, this is "Stage 1"). The four sleep latencies are averaged to give the result, the "mean sleep latency."

question. Each company that produces such a device develops an algorithm, a complex formula using the inputs from the device to decide the sleep stage at any moment. There has been improvement in these devices over the past few years, but it seems unlikely they can ever reach the level of accuracy of in-lab studies, lacking the critical EEG component that feeds into the traditional decision process for sleep stages.

Another sleep study performed in the lab is worth mentioning: the multiple sleep latency test, or MSLT. This is commonly known as a "nap test," and consists of multiple scheduled naps in a single day (usually four or five

	Nap 1	Nap 2	Nap 3	Nap 4	Mean Values
Start time	7:38:43am	9:23:13am	11:19:13am	1:16:43pm	
End time	7:57:13am	9:47:13am	11:42:43am	1:42:13pm	
Time in bed (min)	18.50	24.00	23.50	25.50	22.88
Total Sleep Time (min)	15.50	21.00	16.00	16.00	17.25
Sleep Latency (min)	**3.00**	**3.00**	**7.50**	**9.00**	**5.63**
REM Latency (min)	NONE	NONE	NONE	NONE	

TABLE 1. The numerical part of the sleep technician's report to the interpreting physician of the results of the five-nap MSLT in Table 1 above. The sleep latency (the time it took to fall asleep) is listed in bold for each nap; the mean sleep latency of the average times to fall asleep in each nap is 5.63 minutes, which qualifies as "pathologic sleepiness," as under 8 minutes is considered abnormal.

naps, each separated by two hours of wake) while wearing the full EEG/EOG/EMG setup. The goal is to measure "mean sleep latency," which is simply how many minutes, on average, it takes to fall asleep in those naps.

The MSLT is a test to answer the question: "Why is this person sleepy?" So it's used in situations when regular history, examination, and other tests do not answer that question first. The MSLT Is based on the theory that the sleepier one is, the faster one will fall asleep when given the opportunity, and this test gives multiple opportunities to fall asleep under presumably comfortable and non-stimulating conditions; a normal result would be an average of eight to 15 minutes to fall asleep across all the naps; a result less than eight minutes is considered "pathologic sleepiness" and then leads to further examination to determine the cause.

Pathologic sleepiness as shown on the MSLT may be caused by narcolepsy or another important disorder called "idiopathic hypersomnia," or IHS. We will discuss these in detail later. Both of these illnesses involve sleepiness that comes from the brain itself, so they are called "central hypersomnias." (Hypersomnia means a disorder of excessive sleepiness.) The presence of REM sleep during short naps is abnormal and may indicate narcolepsy. Abnormal REM sleep is always sought on MSLTs as a result, but is not seen in IHS. The slightest hint of REM sleep in any MSLT is important; the absence of any REM favors the diagnosis of IHS. Suspicion of one of these problems is the only reason to use the MSLT in clinical medicine, as it is too labor-intensive and expensive to use for more common causes of daytime sleepiness, like sleep apnea or simple insufficient sleep.

Having learned so much about human sleep from these studies, can we do the same for animals? Insects? Can we even study them?

Giraffes, dolphins, and friends

The study of the sleep of mammals,[16] reptiles, and insects[17] is fascinating unto itself, perhaps even moreso when compared to that of humans. We can draw some conclusions about human sleep if we find similarities in mammals: that is, if we find REM sleep in elephants, we can deduce that REM sleep did not evolve with our species but much further back in the evolutionary tree, before we broke away from elephants and other mammals. If we find it in reptiles or insects, we go even further back down the evolutionary path, towards the actual roots of life on earth. If we could pinpoint when REM sleep (or any other aspect of sleep, or sleep itself) first showed itself, we might have a better grip on the *purpose* of sleep.

So thinking about sleep in mammals, for example, starts, as we have seen, with needing a definition. Can we define "sleep" in animals? How do we know if the animal is asleep? How do we know it isn't just resting, with its eyes closed? If you find yourself standing next to a lion with its eyes closed, it may be useful to be able to tell if it's asleep—or awake, just pondering what a tasty morsel you might be!

It might be easier to be sure when a dog is sleeping, if it's lying down with eyes closed, maybe breathing regularly and slightly noisily, maybe having occasional jerky movements, not responding to mild noises in the environment, or even someone quietly calling his/her name. We're already familiar with the need to have "relative unresponsiveness to the environment" in our definition of sleep, indicating lack of response to milder sounds, and sensations like pain, compared to wakefulness.

And many animals sleep lying down. That makes it easier with a dog or cat or elephant (or lion) to guess if it is asleep, but is perhaps a bit harder with a horse (who sleeps mostly standing), even harder with a snake or, with most difficulty, an insect. How can you ever be sure that a fly on the wall is awake, just resting, or asleep? We can put electrodes on the scalps of larger mammals, and make decisions about REM and non-REM sleep with brainwaves. Harder with a mosquito!

Insects, it turns out, do not have movable eyes (who knew?), but some of the other members of their phylum, the arthropods, do: the jumping spider, for example. REM sleep has been inferred in jumping spiders by noting characteristic eye movements at times when the spider appears to be resting at night, and showing some twitching muscle movements and leg curling, suggestive of sleep.

Eye movements are hard to see in fish, but since zebrafish are transparent when very young, scientists have tagged certain proteins to make them glow, and used a microscope to see a type of glowing protein uptake in nerve cells that suggests REM sleep. This is still controversial. Researchers have now used voltage-sensing dyes[18] to visualize the electrical activity of groups of nerve cells in the fruit fly, and have documented what appears to be deep (that is, delta- or slow-wave) sleep.

Remember how we stage sleep with EEG/EOG/EMG? That is, with measures of brain waves (EEG), measures of eye movements (EOG), and measures of muscle relaxation (EMG)? In captivity, some animals' sleep can be observed with true EEG. And if brain waves aren't available in the smaller beings, we might still infer eye movements (if they have movable eyes), but in the absence of that, those twitches mentioned above, made by mammals in REM sleep (humans too) can help. And back to that fly: if we can't tell if it's resting or sleeping if it doesn't lie down, we might look for "droopiness" or "gravity-related posture" (like the leg-curling in the spider, above) to see if it's relaxed more than in usual wakefulness. This is getting a bit nonspecific, I admit.

Evidence of REM sleep is found in all terrestrial (land-based) mammals, but not in marine mammals like dolphins and whales.[19] They have deep sleep (slow waves) but no REM sleep, and some can sleep while swimming with one half of the brain—one hemisphere—is asleep, showing slow waves, and the other hemisphere awake. A group of swimming dolphins (a pod) can be guarded by the two end dolphins, one on either side, as each has one eye, the one connected to the awake half of the brain, open and maintaining vigilance for predators, the other eye closed. The entire pod may be asleep and continue swimming. Fur seals take this a bit further, swimming with one half of the brain and the flipper on that side asleep, and the flipper on the other, awake-half-brain side doing the propelling. On land, the fur seal sleeps with its full brain, and both flippers are relaxed.

Sleep quotas in mammals used to be thought to vary with size, with the largest animals getting the least sleep (the horse three hours of sleep every 24 hours, the giraffe only two), and the smaller ones the most (bats, 19; possums,18). Mammals in the wild have been shown to sleep even less than in captivity—that makes sense. Out there, they worry more about predators. But it turns out that this sleep-length-to-body-size ratio applies only to herbivores, not to carnivores or omnivores (like man). Why would that be? Other attempts to correlate sleep length or REM amounts with brain size, metabolic rate, or maturity at birth have failed.

We really don't know what determines, in a given species, the amount or character of sleep that species needs.

CHAPTER 2

More Sleep Basics

This is how we do it

Consider a stereotypical sleep pattern. As an adult, one might spend the day awake, maybe for 16 hours, then get sleepy in the late evening, crawl into bed and sleep lying down for 7–8 hours, then awake refreshed, and go back to daily activity. Rinse, repeat. This pattern, common as it might be, is different for different age groups, and even for different individuals. What everyone shares across all groups is the need for sleep, the need for the different stages of sleep, and the need for enough of each of those to make our periods of wakefulness feel like true wakefulness; to be fully alert.

Break this pattern down a bit more (look at **Figure 1,** page 33, the young and older adult versions, for visual reference of this): we get drowsy around the same time every night, maybe doze in a chair (some brief stage N1 [transitional] sleep, maybe even some stage N2 [light] sleep for a few minutes), then wake, brush teeth, undress, get in bed, spend 10–15 minutes awake with eyes closed, then enter sleep in N1, quickly moving into N2 sleep. Depending on many factors (previous night's sleep, previous day's exercise intensity, age, alcohol use, etc.), we may go into deep sleep then, for a few minutes or an hour or more. Then we return to our "baseline" sleep, which is N2.

Perhaps 90–120 minutes after sleep onset, we move into REM sleep: stage R. We almost always enter REM from, and leave REM to, stage N2. Remember REM? We are almost paralyzed, but our brains are busy: more brain activity, more brain blood flow, and 80% of all dreams occur in REM, with more complex plot structures than in non-REM sleep.

We may have more deep (N3) sleep later in the night, or maybe none after that first one. (Younger people have more.) But we will typically continue to cycle back and forth for the last half of the night between REM and N2, with REM occurring every 90–120 minutes and REM periods getting longer as the night goes on. So the predominance of deep sleep is in the first third of the night, and REM tends to be more in the second half. This difference is important in our understanding of some sleep disorders, especially sleepwalking and a rarer one called REM sleep behavior disorder. (See Chapter Six.)

Sleep studies show, in most people, frequent brief awakenings ("arousals") during normal sleep, particularly from N2 sleep (look at **Figure 1** again). These are by definition so brief (a few seconds) that they are not impressed into memory: we have no recall of these then, or the next day. But if we are awakened completely, either by an external stimulus (telephone, car horn, bedpartner snoring, house creaking, and so forth) or from an internal stimulus (need to urinate, pain, a bad dream), our responsiveness then depends on the stage of sleep we are leaving.

If we wake from N2 sleep, our transition may be smooth but brief: a few seconds of lying quietly relaxed, slowly realizing that we are waking, then gradually achieving full wakefulness. If we wake from REM sleep, we may still be emotionally involved in a dream we were just experiencing, and have some detailed memory of it we can relate to our bedpartner. We wake pretty quickly. We sometimes even insert into our dream the stimulus that is waking us: years ago, I once awoke from a dream in which I was searching* for a buzzing sound behind a wall in my house. I remember hammering large ragged holes in the baseboard molding of the

---

* Remember "searching." We will be discussing the presence of searching behaviors in another sleep behavior later: sleepwalking.

wall in my dream, and even today I can still recall the feeling of mounting frustration that I could not find the source of the sound within the walls. Then I awoke to find that my alarm was going off. I was incorporating the sound of the alarm into the plot structure of my dream narrative.

That was an awakening from REM sleep. In contrast, if we are awakened from deep (N3) sleep, it's a different story: we find it difficult to wake, difficult to "kickstart" our brains, to get those slow waves moved up to wake speed, get the diminished brain blood flow and brain temperature of deep sleep up to waking levels. Coming quickly out of deep sleep we may even be confused, able to pick up the phone and answer it, but temporarily unable to identify our situation or the person calling, or to understand the situation prompting the call for a few seconds. This has been described as "sleep inertia," and is a normal aspect of the relationship between deep sleep and stage W (wake).

It can be disturbing to have your mother call you an hour after you have fallen asleep in the evening, and then to find yourself coming too slowly out of deep sleep and unable to recognize her voice or understand why she's calling you for a little bit. But then you get it together, gradually come to perceive your situation, and complete the call (after apologizing for the confusion).

The situation is the same on awakening at our normal wake time in the morning, except that it would be unusual to wake from deep sleep then, as most N3 occurs early in the night, especially in adults. Compare that to waking an adolescent: if you've parented one you know he or she can be difficult—sometimes *very* difficult—to wake after sleep onset and even late in the morning, which fits with our knowledge that adolescents have deep sleep early, as do adults, but even later in the night and even into the morning, unlike adults.

Their growing brains experience more deep sleep during daytime sleep, too, so we can see similar problems with them in waking from a nap. As for adults, we typically wake in the mornings from N2 or REM, and if coming out of REM, we may recall a dream we just exited from, but not any of the other dreams from any other REM periods earlier in the night (unless we woke from those too). This raises the issue of memory and sleep. We sense that there must be a strong connection…and there is.

Thanks for the memories

Lots of studies have focused on how sleep affects memory; the intriguing relation between sleep and immediate memory is worth mentioning. Simply speaking, we must be awake for roughly five minutes *after* an event in order to remember that event later. For example, if my dog barks loudly in my bedroom in the middle of the night and I "arouse" for only a few seconds, but never become fully awake, not surprisingly I will not remember that barking the next morning. If he barks enough to wake me fully and I'm awake for 20 minutes comforting him, I will have no difficulty remembering that experience the next morning.

What is surprising, though, is if I am awake for only three minutes, even if I sit up and comfort him briefly, I will not remember any of that the next morning. The key to this is my rapid return to sleep after the event: most of the time when something disturbing like this occurs at night, the degree of the disturbance affects how easily we can return to sleep after. Only under unusual circumstances would I be able to go back to sleep quickly after a disturbing experience, so usually I will remember it easily later.

Suppose it's routine that I am awakened to pee nightly around 3am (prostate, I'm talking to you). Will I always remember that awakening the next morning, as boring an event as that might be? Experience would say yes, almost always, but then we can postulate that I must therefore be awake for at least five minutes *after* the event to get that experience into memory. If I am so sleepy that I can return to sleep within one to two minutes after getting back into bed, I will not remember that episode the next morning.

Again, we know this is true from studies that measure the exact times to return to sleep after an event of wake. Whenever we are told that something happened during our sleep period that we don't remember, we can reason that we were not awake long enough for the experience to be imprinted into memory. Have you ever awakened in the morning from a dream you remembered, but then dozed again and later found you could no longer remember that wonderful dream? You must have been awake too little time after waking from the dream, so you lost the memory when you returned to sleep.

The Holy Grail of sleep and memory is "sleep learning." If we could listen to those audio tapes from that college course on Western Civilization during sleep for a few weeks and then ace the final exam without ever opening the book during the day, clearly that would revolutionize learning, and change college life forever! But of course, sleep learning has been tried, in different ways, over many years, and has always failed. Otherwise, we would all be doing it today. The visual input for learning is obviously not available during sleep, and the auditory one isn't either, understandable given my reaction to the dog barking during the night described above. An element of minimal wakefulness is required to allow memory of the event.*

But obviously, sleep does impact memory, and therefore learning, as we have just seen. Recent research has shed light on how learning works in the brain: memory of a new event or new data during the day is normally stored short-term in the hippocampus and later moved to the cortex of the brain for longer term storage. This memory of the event degrades over time, but not at first: if there is a period of sleep (as little as two hours) after the event, the memory is strengthened. Selective sleep deprivation studies—waking a person every time they enter N3 (deep) or REM sleep, allowing only sleep without those stages—have suggested that it is during deep sleep (N3) that memory for general knowledge (things we've learned, like the capital of Wisconsin, or "declarative memory") is consolidated in

---

* Researchers have been able to replay memories in the brain by administering auditory (sound) and olfactory (smell) stimuli during sleep, if those same sounds or smells were associated with the initial experience being replayed. Watching brain areas light up on functional MRI with those stimuli is similar to watching rat "place neurons" light up on experience replay, as described below.

the brain, and during REM sleep that non-declarative memory (how to ride a bicycle, say: "procedural memory") is consolidated.*

For some time now students have been encouraged to stay up late to study for an exam and then sleep after, rather than get up early in the morning before the exam to study, as sleep after learning strengthens memory. If you get up early to study before an exam, there is no deep sleep after studying to help consolidate memory of the material, and therefore less likelihood you will recall that studied material for the exam.

REM sleep may also serve to promote retention of *emotional* memories; this makes some sense, if you think of dreams as frequently containing emotional content. We will discuss this further in the section on dreams and emotions.

It is now feasible to study human brain waves *intracerebrally,* that is, with electrodes in direct contact with brain tissue in living humans. This may best be done during neurosurgery† for other problems (typically for resistant epilepsy). It does give a much more direct idea of what the brain is doing at any stage of sleep. Recordings can be taken right from the hippocampus, for example, where new memories are stored, and from many other areas of the brain.

Without getting too technical, I will throw out the names of some waveforms that can be gleaned from surface electrodes and intracellular ones, that are now getting a lot of attention in the study of sleep and memory:

---

* Declarative memory is divided into episodic *memory*, which is of specific events, like last night's dinner, and *semantic memory*, like general information, such as the name of your senator. I like to use the word "declarative" to refer to memories that can be described in words, or "declared." "Non-declarative" memories include procedural memories, and are those that are hard to describe but easy to conceive: for example, I can picture in my mind the elements I have mastered in learning to ride a bike or play ping-pong well, but would have difficulty putting into words all the elements of these procedures. Can you imagine being given the task of writing a brochure of no more than two paragraphs that would teach a novice to ride a bike? And yet you have no difficulty retrieving the learned elements of bike riding that are stored in your long-term memory: "You never forget how to ride a bike."

† That is, the electrodes can be implanted during surgery—with informed consent— and then used to monitor brain activity during sleep some days postoperatively.

PGO waves, K-complexes, sleep spindles, theta waves, and hippocampal "ripples." For years the significance of these waveforms was not understood but now it appears that their appearance correlates with learning, with memory consolidation, in promoting neural plasticity (growth of neural networks).

K-complexes, for example, are short jerky waves on EEG that mark stage N2 sleep. Spindles are short rapid waveforms that appear also during stage N2 sleep; both are thought to strengthen memories. Ripples occur with spindles at times and appear to indicate transfer of memory from hippocampus (short-term storage) to cortex (long-term storage). Slow waves, as in delta sleep, induce synaptic downscaling, or pruning: promoting forgetting. These are some of the ways the brain picks and chooses what to remember and what to forget, and how sleep influences that process.

I think this next finding about sleep and memory is stunning. It starts with rats. Rats[20] in 1984, and now humans[21] have been found to have hippocampal "place neurons." Place neurons are nerve cells that store memory of a particular place, and studies in rats measuring the firing of an individual nerve cell in the rat brain can link up that firing with a particular place in the rat's real-world experience. More specifically, if a rat walks through a maze while nerve impulses are being monitored, place cells for the beginning, middle, and end of the maze are seen to fire in sequence: beginning of the maze, middle, end.

But here's the good part: later, when the rat sleeps in light (N2) sleep, these cells can be seen to fire in the same sequence, as if the rat is retracing its footsteps in the maze during sleep. And it happens over and over, and at *six to 20 times faster* than it occurred in the real maze, which suggests that the rat is reviewing and reviewing and reviewing, at high speed, the path through the maze, for maximal memory consolidation.

The replay occurs not only in the hippocampus, for short-term memory storage, but also in the cortex, which is where longer-term memory is laid down. So the rat is learning, reviewing, and consolidating that memory during sleep, for better retrieval later. This has been shown to be related to the creation as well as the elimination of synapses (the connections between nerve cells): learning during wakefulness—and we can think of all wakefulness as learning, however mundane—increases the strength of synapses throughout the brain, and then during sleep the "nonessential" synapses are weakened or eliminated.

It appears that in REM sleep the older synapses (representing information already sent off to the cortex for long-term storage) in the hippocampus are weakened, which makes those areas of the hippocampus available for new memories in the future. The brain uses a lot of energy (up to 25% of the body's glucose expenditure during wake, though the brain is only 2% of the body's mass), and during sleep, energy appears to be conserved by removing unwanted nerve connections.

More learning during wake promotes more sleepiness; sleep winnows out the nonessential synapses (the unnecessary learning) and strengthens the needed ones. Sleep improves memory and selectively blocks or promotes forgetting.

This occurs with procedural as well as with declarative (data) memory: if two groups are taught a procedure (for example, joystick routines or rapid finger movement tests) and then one group sleeps and the other just rests awake, then, as we might predict, the slept group will perform the procedure better than the rested group. This is the same process of selective strengthening of nerve connections.

The process of building synapses (nerve connections) in the brain during sleep is now understood to be basic to our understanding of brain development during fetal development, infancy, childhood, adolescence, and adulthood. I have alluded to this concept earlier, but now we can formalize it, to a degree. During learning while awake, new synapses are produced (think of them, simplistically, as new data points in our memories, at first in RAM—"rapid access memory," the temporary storage mechanism in a computer—and later on the hard drive, for long-term storage).*

Numerous studies have documented that the brain storage of memories, whether factual (declarative memories) or motor (procedural memories),

---

* One must apologize, at least once, for using the convenient analogy of the brain to a computer. The brain is far more complex (and fascinating), and our understanding of how the brain handles memory is still rudimentary.

is facilitated by sleep; if the memories of procedural performances are tested after a period of sleep, they are stronger than when tested without.

The classic teaching has been that REM sleep stimulates synaptic growth, strengthening new memories, and deep sleep promotes "pruning" of synapses, removing some memories—maybe up to 80%—thereby strengthening the remaining ones and making room for newer memories to be added in the future. This is a tremendously attractive theory, since in infancy and early childhood up to 50% of sleep is in REM (and a form of REM is thought to be present even in fetal development), the period of our lives when rapid brain development is occurring as we are exposed to a myriad of new experiences every day. We are building a vast memory storage system related to all we see, hear, smell, feel, and taste.

In late childhood and getting into adolescence, we begin shifting to larger amounts of stage N3 sleep; teenagers can have multiple long periods of deep sleep every night, and begin to revert to adult amounts of REM sleep (around 25%) in their 20s. In our theory, the pruning that occurs during this time is the brain's big chance to select the important things—experiences, facts, motor movements—to remember, jettisoning others as less important. As this process of brain maturation occurs during sleep, the basic structures of personality and intellect, the foundations of critical thinking, cognition, and reasoning are being built.[*] But when is this process complete? I don't know if there's yet an answer for that. Ask yourself: when did you become a complete adult? Are you even a complete adult now? What is a complete adult?

Beginning around age 40 we see the beginnings of a drop-off in the percentage of deep sleep in normal adults.[†] Are our brains fully built then? There's little reason to think we have stopped making and pruning synapses (our brains still show "plasticity") but just not at the rate seen

---

[*] Some have theorized that mental disorders that make themselves known in adolescence and early adulthood, such as depression, schizophrenia, bipolar disease, and attention deficit disorders, are the results of abnormal non-REM sleep.

[†] This drop-off is a very important concept in understanding sleepwalking. We will discuss this later.

during earlier development. By age 70, we have lost 80% of the nightly deep sleep we experienced when young (but sleep deprivation and exercise can still promote a bump in deep sleep on a given night).

This theory, relegating nerve cell and synapse growth, basically brain growth, to REM sleep and relegating synapse pruning for brain "shaping" and memory consolidation to non-REM sleep, may well be correct, and it is a useful construct to help us understand the changes in normal sleep that occur in our brains as we develop and age, and the importance of sleep in the process of development. Some studies in mice, though, suggest pruning of motor nerve spines (branches) during REM[22] and formation of new nerve cell spines during non-REM sleep.[23]

We can conclude that sleep plays a major role in brain development and learning throughout our lives, and reasoning backwards from our knowledge of the predominance of REM in infancy and childhood and the predominance of deep sleep in adolescence, we know these stages do have distinct and critically different effects on brain development during those different phases within our lives. Matthew Walker wonderfully ponders this in his 2017 book on sleep.[24]

Overall, this process may be the most important function of sleep yet demonstrated. In the next section we'll discuss another remarkable candidate for the "why" of sleep.

Cleanliness is next to...

One of the critical "cleansing mechanisms" in the bodies of mammals is the lymphatic system: a waste-removal system of channels throughout the body that connects the vessels and the organs to lymph channels and lymph nodes; these channels carry off unnecessary or harmful substances, such as products of inflammation, cellular debris, dead bacteria, and products of metabolism. The waste is taken to the liver for recycling or to the kidneys for excretion. All organs in the body have access to the lymphatic system, except the brain—or so it was previously thought. The "blood-brain-barrier," a membrane that surrounds the brain and spinal cord, was thought to be enough to protect the system from most problems; it was thought that the brain did not need a sewage system.

But that theory did not explain how the brain would deal with normal byproducts of its own neurons' metabolism, or the occasional bad thing—a bacterial infection, for example—that would sneak across the blood-brain barrier but then get destroyed. Each cell in the body, neurons included, produces waste as part of the metabolic process, whether producing energy or making proteins. Just as any internal combustion engine has exhaust, all cells produce waste that requires disposal and that can be harmful if it sticks around, piles up, and disrupts local processes. Like garbage collecting on a New York street during a sanitation workers' strike. But until recently, no one knew how the brain could deal with waste.

Then, in 2013, one of the most surprising and exciting findings I have ever learned about sleep was discovered by researchers at the University of Rochester.[25] They found that certain non-nerve brain cells, called glial cells, actually *shrink* in volume, by up to 40%, but only during sleep. There are other cells in the body that can shrink when they need to, such as kidney, fat, and muscle cells, but no one before this knew that these brain cells could make themselves smaller during sleep.

These glial cells line the blood vessels in the brain, and when they shrink they open up channels for *cerebrospinal fluid* (CSF) to flow through the brain, alongside the outside walls of these vessels. CSF is a watery fluid that surrounds the brain and spinal cord. Our concept of CSF dynamics up until this discovery was that the brain and spinal cord were surrounded by CSF, from the bottom of the spinal canal at the base of the spine to the top of the skull, but that the CSF did not penetrate significantly into the substance of the cord or brain.

This new information upended centuries of thought about CSF and its function. The research further showed that, as the CSF flows through the brain (only during sleep, remember), it lowered the concentration of ("washed out," or cleared) certain substances. Now it is apparent how the brain could deal with its waste, how the central nervous system could still connect to the conventional lymphatic system—the waste management system of the body.

This new flow pattern of channels created by glial cells (and acting like lymphatics) around brain arteries and veins merited a new name derived from both names: *the glymphatic system (glial + lymphatic = glymphatic)*. The opening of channels on the outside of arteries allows the pulsations of the arteries to pump the CSF along their walls into the substance of the brain, and the CSF to return alongside large veins, eventually delivering the fluid to the regular lymphatic system at the base of the brain. This circular pattern clears certain metabolic products from the brain, for eventual disposal or recycling just as in the body's conventional system.

So the brain *does* have its own waste-disposal system; we just couldn't see it before 2013.

The next striking thing discovered in 2013 is that the glymphatic system, which operates mainly during sleep, serves to increase clearance from the brain of some important compounds, the most important of which is beta-amyloid. You've probably heard of the protein *beta-amyloid*, it appears to be one of the main culprits behind Alzheimer's, the most common type of dementia worldwide. It is a metabolic (or waste) product of nerve cells, normally not a problem—but in Alzheimer's, it forms into "clumps" among brain neurons, starting early in the hippocampus (the center of memory) and slowly, usually over some years' time, spreading throughout the brain. The finding that the glymphatic system might promote removal and excretion of beta-amyloid from the brain was important in our understanding of that cleansing system; the finding that it occurred mostly during sleep was very important in our understanding of the function of sleep.

There are other proteins that do damage in Alzheimer's, the most important of which is called *tau*. So-called "tau-tangles" are also seen microscopically in the brains of those patients, and studies suggest that the glymphatic system may also promote clearance of tau. The sneaky thing about the deposition of amyloid and tau is that they can both accumulate quietly in the brain in people years before any cognitive decline, suggesting that the lag time between accumulation and disease onset may be long.

A piece of good news: levels of tau can be measured in the blood,[26] and since tau levels seem to correlate with amyloid levels in the brain, we have some optimism that a reliable blood test for Alzheimer's is not far off. If there are "neuroprotective" measures that could be taken in the future to prevent Alzheimer's, a blood test to find those at risk will prove invaluable.

Recently, FDA approval has been sought for a number of new drugs that are aimed at lowering beta-amyloid levels in patients with Alzheimer's; early information has been disappointing, however, suggesting that cognitive function may not improve with these drugs, that attacking beta-amyloid may not reverse this most common form of dementia.

Most important for our understanding of the interaction of sleep and clearance of beta-amyloid is the fact that slow-wave sleep (delta sleep) appears to be the important sleep stage during which the opening of the glial channels, and therefore when most of the clearance of metabolic products during sleep, occurs. Knowing this, we can guess (and it's mostly a guess) that things that increase delta sleep, such as exercise, may benefit our brains by increasing the clearance of beta-amyloid. Recent research[27] has calculated the risk of dementia with the usual decrease in deep sleep with age: 868 people had two sleep studies each, an average of five years apart, and were then followed for 17 years, and the risk of dementia increased by 27% for each decrease of 1% in deep sleep between the two sleep studies. Remember the adage "correlation does not prove causation"? This is an example of where that warning is appropriate.

We know that deep sleep percentages are less in older people, and that dementia increases in older populations, but do we know one causes the other? I can speculate about this, keeping top-of-mind that this is pure speculation: since many of us exercise less as we age, and since exercise is perhaps the most important promoter of deep sleep in adults, might not less exercise be the reason (or one of the reasons) that there is less deep sleep as we age? If so, does the research above mean that more exercise means more deep sleep and therefore less dementia?

This is entirely possible, but by no means proven. Is more exercise better for you as you age? This is suggested by many kinds of studies showing chemical and physical and mental advantages of exercise with age. But again, have we proof that exercise will prevent dementia by increasing deep sleep? There are observational studies suggesting that active exercisers from middle-age onward have 20–40% less risk of dementia. Not proof, but helpful. The perfect study would start with a large group of middle-aged adults, follow their exercise patterns and their deep sleep percentages over, say, 30 or 40 years, then see who develops dementia and who doesn't.

Start that study today and we'll have our answers by 2060. Maybe I can issue a new edition of this book when that happens!

The other main promoter of deep sleep is sleep deprivation, but unfortunately we can't logically prescribe sleep deprivation to lower amyloid levels in the brain, as by definition, sleep deprivation itself should worsen clearance, just from the missing sleep. In fact, experiments in humans[28] using PET scans have shown that *a single night* of sleep deprivation is associated with increased amyloid deposition, especially in the hippocampus.

But before we start panicking each time we miss some sleep, fearing that we may be incurring irreversible brain damage, it's worth reminding ourselves that amyloid deposition is rarely detected in young people and middle-aged people, though many if not most of us have missed sleep at times during our youth, sometimes large amounts. How reversible are the amyloid effects from one night or many nights of insufficient sleep? If each night of sleep deprivation in the early decades of our lives resulted in irreversible amyloid deposition, might we not expect many more cases of Alzheimer's in middle age than now exist?

Does this concern, that missing sleep may predispose to amyloid deposition, lead us to conclude that we should be taking sleeping pills ("hypnotics") to ensure that we never miss sleep? We will be discussing sleeping pills in the sections on insomnia, but for now, let's think about them knowing what we know about the glymphatic system. Let's start with some assumptions.

First, assume that there may be a subjective benefit to clearing metabolic products from the brain as occurs during sleep; in other words, that one of the main reasons we feel good on awakening is due to having a "cleaner brain" as a result of the glymphatic clearance of lots of metabolic products we experienced during slow-wave sleep.

Second, assume that we are sampling a number of sleeping pills, which are pharmaceutical products that are taken orally, by prescription or over-the-counter, and that these drugs produce sleepiness by a number of different mechanisms. For example, some work by inhibiting histamine, which is an alerting neurotransmitter in the brain. These are antihistamines, some of which have a strong sleepiness effect. Others work by blocking orexin, another alerting neurotransmitter, and some by promoting the effects of GABA, which inhibits nerve transmission in the brain and thereby promotes sleepiness. Still others work by imitating melatonin, or as a side-effect of sleepiness occurring incidentally in antidepressant medications. More on this in the section on insomnia.

However these hypnotics work, we ask: do they help people sleep? That answer appears to be yes, for most people. They tend to result in a few more minutes of sleep in normal subjects per night. Do they make people feel better the next morning? Again, for most people, yes, but maybe with some side effects like grogginess in the morning, and with some tolerance (benefits diminishing after continued use). Then we ask: what is the *quality* of the sleep that occurs with these pills? Do they promote deep sleep, the sleep that seems most restorative subjectively, the sleep that promotes clearance of metabolic products from the brain?

It turns out that most hypnotics do not promote delta sleep; they tend to suppress it, while increasing stage N2 and REM sleep more. One antidepressant that does tend to increase delta sleep and is used off-label (without a formal FDA indication for insomnia) is trazodone. Trazodone is the favored hypnotic prescribed by many primary care physicians, and many insomnia patients find it helpful. But does this mean it has its effect through delta sleep by improving amyloid clearance? That it reduces dementia risk or even prolongs life by forestalling or preventing Alzheimer's? One could break a very large leg in jumping to such conclusions.

To find an hypnotic that perfectly mimics normal sleep is to find the Holy Grail of sleeping pills.

Sleeping pills comprise the largest selling group of drugs in the world, and yet their use has significant drawbacks. The development of a sleeping pill that induces *natural* sleep—with normal amounts of all stages of sleep—would be earthshaking... and profitable. This new drug should promote lots of deep sleep and lots of glymphatic flow (and lots of N2 and REM sleep to promote learning). We could go so far as to hope that this drug would lower the risk of Alzheimer's over time. It is devoutly to be wished. My fingers are crossed.

Lots more on sleeping pills later. Let's explore now what happens when we can't, or won't, get enough sleep.

I'm so tired, I haven't slept a wink

In 1879 Thomas Edison announced the invention of the first successful electric light bulb. Admittedly, he had tried hundreds of variations on this bulb before, and others were making progress on this discovery at the same time, but Edison gets the credit—which may not be all good. Why? Because, it has been claimed, the worst thing that ever happened to human sleep was the introduction of the electric light bulb. You will see that is not an unreasonable claim.

Of all the sleep disorders we deal with in sleep medicine, of all the things that can go wrong with our sleep, it appears that *sleep deprivation*, or insufficient sleep, is the most common. This means, simply, not getting enough sleep. We defined normal sleep earlier as "sleep with the right quality and quantity to allow normal alertness, normal body functioning, and normal mood the following day," so we can then say "enough" normal sleep is "enough to feel and think well the following day." Remember that meta-study [29](compilation of previous studies) that concluded that seven hours was the minimal amount of sleep required? Let's use this as our standard, admitting that some can do well on less.

Now we have a reference point for what is and what isn't enough sleep; sleep length less than seven hours in most people is insufficient sleep, and less than six hours nightly is clearly insufficient sleep for almost everyone. Surveys show that 28–45% of Americans average less than seven hours of sleep nightly.[30] We all know reasons why that might be: high among them are work and family demands. But the brain demands sleep just as the body demands food and water, and the consequences of denying those demands are real.

These results fall into short-term and long-term penalties for the brain being denied the states of unconsciousness it requires. Some of the short-term effects are obvious, some not: difficulty with alertness, attention, and focus, worsening as the day goes on; moodiness and irritability that might not represent our usual personality; and difficulty with reasoning and calculation. We may not be aware we are short-tempered and grouchy when we're chronically sleep-deprived and may not know our reasoning and logic are faulty.

Sleep loss results in a rebound in stage N3 (slow-wave, or deep) sleep.[31] In Chapter One, we mentioned that there are two reliable ways to increase deep sleep: exercise and sleep restriction.* It's no surprise that part of the recovery from sleep deprivation, in the laboratory or at home, is an increase in deep sleep. It's a way of clawing back some of what has been lost. The amount of "rebound" deep sleep may increase for several nights after sleep loss.

Some tests that are used to quantify sleep loss and recovery are standard sleep studies, standardized sleepiness scales (questionnaires), digit symbol substitution tests (DSST), and psychomotor vigilance tests (PVT). The DSST is a timed test of the ability to write, with pencil on paper, a symbol from a table that corresponds to each of 125 different digits; this is meant to be boring and tedious and is a standardized way of measuring alertness and attention. The PVT measures reaction times as the ability to push a button repeatedly in response to random lights on a screen; scores of lapses in button-pushes indicate loss of attention

---

* We will see in Chapter Three that inflammation can promote deep sleep, and that inflammation and sleep deprivation are linked. Alcohol also increases deep sleep, but to the detriment of REM sleep. Not a good tradeoff.

or vigilance. Again, these tests are considered effective in relation to the tedium that they inspire, as vigilance requires a conscious effort to overcome boredom and stick to the task at hand.

For short-term sleep loss (a few nights of short sleep), the amount of recovery sleep needed to reverse all deficits is not completely clear; even when good sleep is restored, the sleepiness (measured by sleep studies and/or standardized sleepiness scales) may improve but the performance issues may persist. One study[32] simulated a workweek with bad sleep (six hours a night for six nights) followed by a recovery weekend, in this case three nights of 10 hours in bed.* Sleepiness improved to baseline after recovery, but performance measures did not. There were persistent lapses in vigilance despite seemingly adequate recovery, present after the third night of prolonged sleep opportunity.

For anyone who hopes that weekend "make-up" sleep will normalize a previous week of poor sleep, this suggests it will not, and this has implications particularly for those in safety-critical careers, such as those in healthcare, heavy machinery operation, piloting, driving, and so forth. And if, after this hypothetical work week, there are persistent behavioral deficits, one can expect these only to worsen if subsequent weeks follow the same pattern of short sleep on work nights followed by attempted but insufficient recovery sleep.

Another study[33] used three weeks of week-night sleep loss with weekend makeup over three weeks. Subjects slept four hours a night for five nights, then eight hours a night for two nights, all repeated three times. Stress hormones[†] were measured intravenously and well-being was assessed with questionnaires. Not too surprisingly, the subjects seemed

---

* Admittedly, not a typical 7-day work week. Also, consider that 10 hours in bed does not necessarily mean 10 hours of sleep: just because I'm sleepy and have the opportunity for 10 hours of sleep doesn't mean I can sleep that long. Circadian factors (trying to sleep past my usual wake time, for example) may interfere with that.

† They measured cortisol and white blood cell interleukin-6.

to accommodate to this short sleep pattern, and by Week Three they said they felt they were subjectively near baseline.

But the stress hormone (cortisol) levels were elevated at Week Two and higher at Week Three, suggesting ongoing inflammation related to accumulated sleep loss. (This fits with the bidirectional nature of sleepiness and inflammation we discussed in the last chapter.) The authors concluded that we may get used to considerably insufficient sleep and not be aware of ongoing inflammatory problems.

What might these "inflammatory problems" cause? Large studies have shown a U-shaped curve for mortality around a seven-to-eight-hour sleep habit, meaning that those (adults) who sleep less than seven *and those who sleep more* than eight hours have a higher mortality—that is, they do not live as long as those with "normal" sleep length. In addition, recall that there is statistically more heart disease, glucose intolerance (pre-diabetes), and even cancer in the long-term short sleepers.[34] If these patterns are true, then there are obviously aspects of sleep that are healthy and, when missed, have consequences, and we may infer that ongoing inflammation may play a role in that.

Here is a problem with sleep studies with large numbers of subjects over long periods of time: the more subjects observed and the longer the study goes on, the more likely it is that sleep amounts are *self-reported*, and less likely that sleep is measured directly, as in a lab. This leaves room for doubt about the accuracy of the sleep times. Self-reported values in all research can be affected by reporting bias, with the subjects more likely to report what they think they are "expected" to report. (This bias is particularly a problem in dietary research in large groups.)

Similarly, the "purity" of the results depends on the exclusion of other confounding effects. For example, it's believed that those who sleep more than nine hours a night have a higher mortality—they don't live as long as those who sleep less. But is this a "pure" study group? Have those who are chronically or seriously ill, and who sleep more as a result of illness, been excluded from the results? Anything that causes longer sleep times (sleeping pills, anyone?) can muddy the conclusion that longer sleep means shorter life. So, we take results like these with a grain of salt—until a more "perfect" study comes along.

Back to Edison: Why was the light bulb's discovery a problem? Because the effect of "light anytime, light all the time" is bad for sleep. Remember our discussion of the onset of darkness stimulating the output of melatonin, with resultant sleepiness? This doesn't happen in the presence of bright electric light in the evening, at least until it is turned off.

Simplistically, bright light tells us, "The sun is up! Be awake!" even at 10pm, and if we require a period of dim light (or darkness) to promote sleepiness, there may not be time before we are impinging on our needed sleep period, resulting in short sleep. If we then sleep later in the mornings, we may begin to reset our circadian rhythms, pushing our timing mechanism to a "later bedtime, later wakeup" pattern that's hard to reverse.

Lights on in the bedroom all night? Even worse. Try this experiment: in the dark, close your eyes while touching the switch of the only lamp in a room. Now turn on the lamp, keeping your eyes closed, and then turn it off again. Could you tell when it was turned on, even though your eyes were closed? Of course you could. In fact, the eyelids do not block all the light from outside, so some still makes it to the retina and from there to the brain, to inhibit sleep.

I may not be able to remove all light from making it into my bedroom at night—the small LED lights from some electronics (that I haven't put duct-tape on), the neighborhood lights that stay on all night—but I do the best I can. Light pollution nationally is getting a lot of attention as a disruptor of nature's rhythms, so at least I can try to minimize the light pollution I am exposed to inside my room during my intended sleep period.

Our understanding of the interaction between light and mood has advanced considerably. Researchers now believe that we need a daily dose of "photons" (the name for the units that light comes packaged in) and a daily dose of darkness to maintain normal circadian rhythms, as we previously discussed, but just as importantly to maintain mood. For quite some time we've recognized that "seasonal affective disorder" (appropriately shortened to "SAD") is a problem with depression that some people experience during times of shorter days and longer nights, which means especially in northern climes in both hemispheres, and in the winter months. And we have known that light therapy—the exposure to bright light, especially in the mornings—can make this depression better.

It is not surprising, then, that more severe depression can improve with better light/dark management. Again, the "doses" are important. Getting more bright light in the mornings, especially direct exposure to sunlight, without sunglasses means getting a higher "photon dose" or dose of light that indoor lighting cannot supply, neither the amount nor the wavelengths available from the sun. A good 30 minutes will do. *Light boxes* are almost as good, as long as they deliver 10,000 lux (the brightness index). Evening bright light is discouraged, though, given that it affects circadian rhythms and may make going to sleep at a normal time more difficult.

Recommendations for sunlight in the mornings can be difficult to follow for those of us who get up before sunrise so we can get to work on time. This is where the light boxes really shine (sorry); a full dose may be absorbed during dressing and morning hygiene, as the light is usually aimed from the side rather than directly at the face, allowing normal activity. There are also *light glasses* that provide a similar function.

And what about that dose of darkness mentioned above? It is said to be equally as important for depression as the light dose, and independent too—meaning that each can help with depression whether the other is there or not, though together they will do their best work. A "good" darkness means really dark, eliminating as much light leaking into the sleep space as possible: not only moonlight or outside night lighting, but also lights from inside the bedroom, such as those in clocks, electronics and nightlights. A diligent search for "light leakage" and a diligent approach to stemming it—which can involve curtains and even a sleep mask—can result in "perfect darkness," which in theory is a light dose of zero.

What about the rest of the world, the nondepressed? Do we need to ramp up our morning daily light dose and get really obsessional about our nightly dark dose? That's not really clear yet, but I suspect we might all benefit from this, maybe achieving better overall mood and sleep. It's worth a try.

A hunger for sleep

Let us now consider the effects of sleep loss on the gastrointestinal system.

There are good data supporting the premise that chronically insufficient sleep increases the risks of weight gain, obesity, and diabetes.[35,36] Consistently sleeping less than seven hours nightly increases risk of obesity by 45%; sleeping less than six hours or even less nightly increases diabetes risk by 28%. These are not small amounts.

When we contemplate sleep and the body's endocrine system—the hormones it uses to keep itself in chemical balance—there are lots of hormone candidates to consider, more than 50 recognized hormones in humans. Hormone output can vary based on sleep or wake, that is, can be controlled by behavior, by when we choose to sleep or not, or they may vary in relation to the clock time, with the day/night cycle, meaning with circadian rhythm.

We can get an overview of this by confining our discussion to three particular hormones. The first is *leptin*, a satiety hormone which is released from adipose (fatty) tissue. Experiencing satiety means feeling *sated*, feeling full, no longer hungry. Leptin gives the signal to stop eating.

The second hormone is *ghrelin,* a hunger (appetite)-promoting hormone that comes from cells in the stomach. Ghrelin tells the body to feel hunger, to eat more.

And the last is *2-AG,** part of the endocannabinoid (eCB) system, a group of hormones that come from different tissues (muscle, pancreas, brain, adipose, and others). The eCBs control feeding, body weight, and interestingly promote "hedonic feeding," which means eating for pleasure. This seems logical when we consider that endocannabinoids are

---

* An abbreviation for 2-arachidonoylglycerol. Don't memorize this.

home-grown hormones that connect with the same receptors as does cannabis (marijuana), a plant form of cannabinol, which increases appetite in a pleasurable way, a sensation that is popularly called "the munchies."

Leptin levels—satiety levels—slowly rise during the day and fall overnight. Rising leptin levels inhibit hunger; this translates to an increased degree of feeling sated, of feeling "full" during the day, and feeling less full overnight. Given normal eating patterns during the day and normal fasting overnight, it makes sense that leptin levels increase all day, and fall during the night when there is no eating.

Ghrelin levels, a more direct influence on increasing appetite, fall sharply after meals, but rise again before the next meal and show a gradual decrease during sleep. The effects of these two hormones together add up to more hunger before meals and on awakening from a normal amount of sleep, and less hunger after eating.

How do these hormones affect appetite after sleep restriction? The studies are conflicting, with some suggesting a drop in leptin levels (more appetite) after prolonged sleep restriction (many nights, as opposed to one night); some suggest that ghrelin (more hunger) may increase with even short-term sleep loss. Other studies have shown no effect. Sleep loss also increases 2-AG levels, causing endocannabinoid effects. These data support the suggestion that more appetite, possibly with more eating for pleasure, results from insufficient sleep, especially if it is chronic.

What are more helpful are studies of subjective hunger combined with measures of food intake when subjects are sleep-deprived. Averaged data[37] from a group of studies confirmed more hunger and a higher than baseline caloric intake (more than 250 calories per person) after chronic sleep loss. There was significantly more weight gain and insulin resistance (pre-diabetes) with insufficient sleep. Late evening snacking was more frequent. The general rule is: "sleepiness makes you hungrier."

We can now speculate that chronically insufficient sleep has a profound influence on metabolism. Beginning in the early 1990s, an "obesity epidemic" arose in America (and has subsequently spread around the developed world). In the US, state by state, the percentages of those

Hormone	Source	Function	Effect of Sleep Loss
Leptin	Adipose (fat) tissue	Satiety hormone: signals fullness, decreases appetite	↓ Leptin → ↓ Satiety → ↑ Appetite
Ghrelin	Stomach	Hunger hormone: signals need to eat, more appetite	↑ Ghrelin → ↑ Hunger
2-AG	Multiple tissues (endocannabinoid system)	Promotes pleasure-based (hedonic) eating	↑ 2-AG → ↑ Pleasure-based eating

TABLE 2. Appetite hormones affected by sleep. Just a few of the many hormones that affect appetite and vary with sleep loss. This represents one mechanism that explains the increase in appetite seen with sleep deprivation.

with mild obesity (BMI*> 30), moderate (BMI > 35) and severe (BMI > 40) rose dramatically into the 2000s, and the prevalence of type 2 diabetes rose proportionately. Now nationally over 40% of adults in America are obese, and obesity is associated with more diabetes, heart disease, stroke, sleep apnea, and some cancers.

The Obesity Epidemic—and that is in fact what it is—has many explanations, none of which is entirely satisfactory. Poor diet (high calorie, high fat, high carbohydrate, lots of preservatives, ultra-processed foods) combined with less exercise, is usually blamed. Was there a huge increase in bad diets in the early 90s that can be blamed? High fructose corn syrup is a major source of carbohydrate intake in the USA, and has been thought to be one of the causes of increasing high-sugar content in our diets. But it's not clear if there was a major increase in its use then.

We're all aware of the increase in screen-viewing time that has swept into our population in the last few decades, with more cell phone and computer use; perhaps this can explain the drop-off in exercise in all age groups. It's widely accepted that children spend more time on video games

---

* *Body mass index*, or BMI, is calculated by dividing body weight in kilograms by the square of the height in meters (BMI = kg/m^2). There is continued search for a more perfect reflection of obesity, but BMI remains a standard measure in sleep medicine.

indoors now and less time playing outside. Poverty, racism, and food insecurity do not explain the obesity rates in all socioeconomic levels.

It's tempting to look at what we just reviewed regarding sleep habits and their relation to appetite, weight gain, obesity, diabetes, and the downstream effects of those (hypertension, heart disease, and cancer) and wonder if sleep insufficiency is not playing a significant role in the Obesity Epidemic. Sleep extension studies (testing subjects with insufficient sleep by promoting longer sleep times) show reversal of some indicators of early diabetes; we in sleep medicine have long advised our patients that a weight loss program is unlikely to be successful unless an improvement in sleep habits is included in the regimen.

The causes of the Obesity Epidemic remain a mystery. Barring some unexpected element being proven to be the cause (such as microplastics in our food, water causing endocrine dysfunction, or widespread exposure to pesticides), we are left with the multifactorial explanations as above. All are addressable (better diet, more exercise), and more sleep should clearly also be a part of that solution.

So sleep affects hunger, and hunger affects sleep. Another important determinant of sleep—perhaps the most important one of all—is light. This has broad and far-reaching effects… especially for the elderly.

Rage against the light

Recall the term "zeitgeber" from Chapter One: a timing signal. Light is the most important zeitgeber for maintaining our circadian rhythms close to a precise 24 hours. This means light is the strongest *timing cue* determining when we should sleep and when we shouldn't. In fact, that first burst of bright light we get in the morning is the most important rhythm-resetting stimulus, and it turns out that of all the colors in the visible light spectrum, blue light has the strongest effect on our circadian system.*

* Light in the yellow-green spectrum has a smaller effect.

The Celestial Design System seems to have arranged that sunlight, for millennia, has reached the surface of our planet having its broad spectrum light (all the colors) broken up by particulate matter in the atmosphere, filtering out much of the spectrum but allowing blue light to get through. ("Is that why the sky is blue, Daddy?" "Yes, Virginia, it is.") We have adapted through evolution to react best to blue light.

Older people have it rough when it comes to light management, in two situations: cataracts and nursing homes. We know that seniors may not have as robust a response to timing cues as younger people, and to keep their circadian patterns firm, to keep them from drifting, they need good light stimuli too, especially blue light.

But blue light in the light spectrum is close to *ultraviolet,* or *UV* (a word which loosely means "very blue"), and UV light has ionizing qualities: it can damage tissue—and even DNA—just as radiation does. In fact, it's the same thing: UV light is a form of radiation. And it's the UV light from sun exposure during daylight that, over a lifetime, is absorbed by our lenses in our eyes, and depending on our genetic predisposition, causes progressive opacities on the lenses which we call cataracts.

Blue light itself is *not* ionizing; damage to retinal cells in animals and in cell cultures has been suggested in research, but is not proven in humans.[38] "Blue-blocking" sunglasses are marketed as protectors of the eyes, preventing "eye-strain" or "sleep problems," but in fact if we don't get blue light in the mornings our circadian rhythms are less stimulated, which potentially could cause sleep timing issues. We need blue light, especially in the mornings. The elderly need it in the evenings.

The American Academy of Ophthalmology does not recommend blue-blocking glasses,[39] and I agree. These glasses do not prevent problems related to radiation (that requires UV-blocking, which all glasses do), so they don't prevent cataracts (or macular degeneration—which is a serious form of retinal damage—the relation of which to UV radiation is less clear. The only times you want to block blue light is at bedtime or during the night, when blue light would be alerting and prevent sleep. For that reason, some digital tablets and phones have a blue-blocking option to be used then. This can help the middle-of-the-night reader to avoid difficulties returning to sleep.

Back to cataracts. The surgical treatment for cataracts is lens replacement: the old, damaged human lens is removed by an ophthalmologist and replaced with an artificial one. Most people need to have both eyes done in sequence, so they have two new lenses implanted sequentially. Most of these synthetic lenses are manufactured to block blue light, but this seems counterproductive, as we just discussed: blocking blue light doesn't prevent eye damage from UV light and may interfere with circadian rhythms. It makes sense to me to have new lenses that transmit blue light normally, and in fact that is what I requested when I had that surgery some years ago. One just has to ask.

If an elderly person does receive new artificial lenses that block out blue light, they are now relatively deprived of blue light as a timing cue in the mornings (and the rest of the day), and they may be missing some of the normal resetting of their circadian rhythm each day. Their set points for waking and sleeping may drift. This may be a contributor to a circadian rhythm problem seen in the elderly called "advanced sleep phase syndrome", which means uncontrollably early sleep and wake times. We will discuss this further in Chapter Four.

Suffice it to say that I recommend avoiding blue-blocker artificial lenses in cataract surgery.

All artificial lenses are UV blockers. They don't develop opacities from exposure to UV light, so no cataracts can recur in the new lenses. They do block most of that UV passing through the lens though, so little UV makes it to the back of the eye, and the chance of retinal damage is small. For the rest of the world, for everyone else that still has their own natural lenses, it does make sense, when out in the sun, to wear sunglasses that are UV-blockers, as most of them are.

A second problem with light management the elderly have is in nursing homes. Traditionally nursing homes are maintained with fairly dim lighting throughout the day, apparently with the understanding that old folks need encouragement to sleep whenever they can. But those old folks need circadian stimulation (zeitgebers) to get the daily reset of their rhythm in nursing homes as well, so it's bright light in the mornings that they need, and bright light in the mornings may help them to be more alert and enjoy their lives during the day, and to sleep better at night.

Herein lies a bit of a problem. That morning bright light helps with timing but, in the elderly, evening bright light makes even more sense. That advanced sleep phase that the elderly shift into (after an adulthood of "normal" circadian rhythm) means they develop a tendency to fall asleep earlier in the evening and to awaken early in the mornings: their rhythm is "advanced" to earlier phases of sleep and wake. The best way to bring that back to normal is with bright light *in the evening,* which delays the sleep phase and allows them to stay up later, and awaken later.

As in any institution, however, this may not work well with staff schedules and food delivery times that are keyed to an older population. If you are the administrator of a large nursing home, you may need to limit variability of meal delivery times to fit the natural tendencies of your populace, so it may be harder to accommodate those elderly who do not want their dinners at 5:30pm. Also, a sleeping nursing home resident is less demanding on staff time than a wakeful one.

A visitor to any nursing home may be impressed to see how many of the residents appear to sleep all day in their chairs in the dayroom. This could be the effect of chronic illness; or the prolonged effects of sleeping pills requested by, or encouraged upon, the patients to permit nighttime sleep; or the side effects of their daily medications; a lack of exercise; or, for some, the sheer boredom of living in a nursing home.

But another important consideration is the lighting environment the seniors are exposed to night and day, as a robust circadian rhythm (as stimulated by more bright light in the mornings and bright light particularly in the evenings) might promote better sleep and better daytime alertness.

Some or all those elderly people you see sleeping during the day in the nursing home may be suffering from dim-light-induced circadian rhythm disruption. More progressive nursing home administrators understand this and have improved the lighting for this vulnerable population.

And-a one and-a two

If we in the 21st century are vulnerable to exposure to electric and other forms of artificial light, does that mean that our sleep patterns are artificial? That if we reverted to an older, pre-electric time, would we sleep differently? Hard to know. In prehistoric times, things were pretty dark before the discovery of fire, obviously, and we don't know much about sleep then. After fire was discovered and particularly after the development of candles and gas lighting, more activities during the dark hours were possible, but brightness of candles and gaslights and lanterns was much less that of electric bulbs, so we can guess that the effects on circadian rhythms these might have caused would be… less.

Could you still stay up all night sitting close to a candle trying to finish reading that last exciting episode of *David Copperfield*? Of course. But in general we would think that before the 19th century people slept more during the dark hours and less during the daylight ones. Did they get more sleep overall than we do? Maybe. Was their sleep pattern different? Maybe.

Maybe they slept in two main periods, rather than just one, as most of us do.

Sleeping in two periods is called *biphasic sleep*, so more modern sleep, all in one period, is monophasic. We promote monophasic sleep as the most restful: "I slept straight through the night last night. I feel great!" And it's reasonable to think that we have "evolved" or "accommodated" to this pattern of sleep such that now it's commonplace and "normal." It certainly seems to work for lots of people.

For those who sleep in two periods of sleep each night, there can be a memorable difference between what we call "first sleep" and "second sleep." You may notice this when waking in the morning after two phases of sleep, if you have experienced involuntary wakefulness in the middle of the night for some external reason. You are aware on awakening in the morning that the second phase felt *different* from the first one: the second felt *deeper*, more *involved*, with more dreams. This is not surprising: remember that most of our "deep" sleep (N3) is in the first third of the night, and most of our REM sleep in the last half.

Remember also that N2 ("light" sleep) is the predominant phase for the whole night. So first sleep is mostly N2 with a sprinkle of N3, and second sleep is N2 with a lot (maybe 40–50%) REM. And if you didn't wake directly from N3 in first sleep, you won't feel the sleep drunkenness that comes from that, just a smoother transition to wake that comes out of N2. But for some reason, waking from second sleep feels heavier after a phase of concentrated REM than first sleep does, even heavier than after waking from normal REM in a one-phase night. Not sure why.

Biphasic sleep isn't that uncommon even now. Many of us nap daily, so we have two phases of sleep, just not both phases in the dark hours. Many people wake (and complain of waking) in the middle of the night, stay awake for an hour or more, then return to sleep. Others don't have those awakenings, and why should they? But is it possible this harkens back to the pre-industrial era (and perhaps many centuries before that) when "normal" sleep may have been biphasic? Have our artificial light systems and our post-industrial lifestyles suppressed biphasic sleep? More questions than answers.

And what about napping? How is napping not biphasic sleep? Does it matter if we try to link two major periods of sleep together as biphasic and say a nap is different because it occurs so long after, or before, the major sleep period of the night? Let's assume that it doesn't matter if one sleeps from 10pm to 1am and then again from 3am to 8am (that would be typical "biphasic sleep"), or overnight from 10pm to 5am and then again in the afternoon from 1pm to 2pm (that would be a conventional "nap"). Would the quality of the sleep at nap time (the makeup of that sleep, i.e., the stages achieved) be comparable to that of the second half of a biphasic sleep time? Should we worry that sleep time taken from a nap during the day will subtract from the quantity (and thereby the quality) of overnight sleep?

In 2006 Sara Mednick wrote a wonderful monograph[40] on napping which would support our assumption that nap quality can be as good as overnight sleep. She contends that daytime nap time does not subtract from nocturnal sleep time (unless the nap is so late in the evening that it inhibits falling asleep at the usual bedtime), and, more importantly, that a nap can be tailored to reap different benefits. She emphasizes that the drive for REM sleep is still active after waking in the morning (that is, the propensity for REM sleep in the second half of the night is still present some hours after awakening), so REM may appear even in a late morning nap.

Similarly, knowing that the drive for sleep is lowest on awakening in the morning (in fact, it should be zero if adequate sleep was obtained the night before), we can say that the drive for deep sleep builds up during the day and makes it more likely to appear in a mid- or especially late-afternoon nap. She goes so far as to "prescribe" naps for people depending on their goals: a morning nap if they are attempting to increase creativity and complex associative memory, by emphasizing REM sleep, or an afternoon nap if slow wave sleep is perceived to be helpful, say for tissue repair (in those with physically demanding jobs) or improved memory recall.

Historians have uncovered evidence[41] of biphasic sleep as early as the 1500s, not only in Europe but in all continents of the world, and at high latitudes (where nights are longer in winter, for example) as well as low ones. A typical sleep pattern in the pre-industrial (pre-artificial light) era in Europe would entail going to sleep at 9pm or 10pm (well after sunset) but waking again two to three hours later and being awake for an hour or more, doing household chores, tending to family, having sex, visiting friends, even working outside in moonlight. One might then return to sleep until dawn or after.

Studies of isolated, primitive cultures in different parts of our modern world have shed light (sorry!) on sleep patterns of modern peoples not exposed to artificial illumination. The results go both ways. Tribes in South America and in West Africa have shown evidence of biphasic sleep, but studies of other tribes in similar regions exhibit monophasic sleep.[42] As well, sleep lengths in these latter tribes were not longer than in ours in the developed world, suggesting that a "normal" sleep response to sunrise and sunset may not have changed much over the centuries. The supposition that primitive man would go to bed at sundown and get up at sunup, in the absence of artificial stimuli, may not be correct.

We admit that we do not have a firm grasp on the definition of normal sleep. We think of pre-industrial sleep—sleep uninhibited by artificial light, television, the internet, and other modern conveniences and interruptors—as being "natural sleep." It might be easier to think of biphasic sleep as a normal variant of sleep, perhaps a tendency that we all retain in our DNA but do not exhibit for social and environmental reasons, because our social and work lives do not offer opportunities for activity in the middle of the night, and our environments, with entertainments and other distractions, fill our wake hours easily without leaving room for more wake in the middle of the night.

Barring the apocalypse, it's unlikely we'll ever revert to a civilization without these influences; at the very least, knowledge of our history of biphasic sleep may offer some solace to those experiencing periods of otherwise-normal mid-sleep wakefulness… as well as to those who just prefer to sleep that way.[43]

Another remarkable aspect of sleep we may never get a firm grasp upon is dreaming.

Mr. Sandman, bring me a dream

Nothing in sleep medicine is more fascinating than the study of dreaming. In some ways it is an unreachable realm of science: one cannot now, and probably never will be able to watch, like a video, someone else's dreams as they sleep. (The closest we come now is watching a mouse's place neurons (see page 71, "Thanks for the memories,") as he retraces his steps in a maze, but who knows what he's actually dreaming?)

The traditional way to do dream research is to watch subjects in a sleep laboratory with polysomnography, monitoring sleep stages, and then to awaken them after a predetermined time or in a particular observed sleep stage and ask them to describe what they are dreaming. About 80% of dreams occur during REM sleep, so 20% or so occur in non-REM sleep (N2 and N3). Dreams in non-REM are said to be with limited plot structure and emotional content, while dreams in REM are more complicated, colorful, and emotional.

Theories of dreams and their meanings go back centuries but were first described most memorably in the modern era by Freud[44] in 1913. He believed that all dreams, whether pleasurable or not, were manifestations of unfulfilled wishes in the subconscious mind. After the first descriptions of REM sleep in 1953 and the subsequent association of dreams with that sleep stage, dreams were re-considered as probably random neuronal activity from the brainstem.

More recent theories, perhaps not surprisingly, relate dreaming to what we have learned about sleep and memories. You recall from our earlier discussions of memory that spindles and ripples in stage N2 sleep are associated with strengthening hippocampal memory short-term storage and transferring data to the cortex for long-term storage, and that deep (N3) sleep is associated with weakening of presumably unwanted memories. REM sleep is associated with emotional memories and creative problem solving, and some motor memories as well.

Dream research does show more emotional content in dreams arising from REM sleep than from non-REM, and such dreams are also more vivid and plot-driven. Dreams in non-REM sleep are simpler and are more likely associated with episodic memories (recent or past events and experiences), though fragments of these occur in REM sleep dreams as well. Past events are not dreamt in their original form, but elements of past experiences can be identified in some dreams. We've all had these dreams, with someone we knew from the past or some past experience entwined into new people or events that make up a weird dream. (Is "weird dream" a tautology? Or redundant? Aren't they all?)

Video games used in dream research show how past and recent experiences can merge in dreams. Of a group of subjects taught to play a video game for the first time, some will go on to incorporate elements of the game in their subsequent dreams. When those who had had prior experience with the game are studied, however, dream analysis shows elements of prior versions of the game in the current dreams, as well as elements from the game used in the study, indicating that the dreamer pulls in more remote experience as well as recent experience into the content of the dreams. What's clear is that it is *not* clear how the brain chooses what experiences and what information to put to the screenplays that make up our dreams.

Functional MRI (fMRI) studies can highlight sections of the brain that are active during sleep and dreaming, and interviews in the MRI scanner after awakenings from certain sleep stages help us understand the brain networks that affect dreams. Regions of the brain involved with processing emotions, like fear or threat, are active during non-REM as well as in REM sleep.

If you ever took Psychology 101, you may remember the concepts of *stimulus reinforcement and extinction.* Simply speaking, anything that strengthens a response to a repeated stimulus is said to reinforce that response; for example, saying "Sit" to your dog may elicit the sitting response, and this response will be reinforced (become more likely to occur as intended) if a treat is given after the desired response. The treat strengthens the response.

On the other hand, extinction allows the response to weaken or die; withholding the treat or speaking harshly to the dog despite her sitting will make her good responses less likely, and even wither over time.

One theory of dreams is that negative emotions (situations, persons, memories) are processed and "learned" in the safer context of a dream (as opposed to in reality) and therefore disconnected from the associated negative outcomes (embarrassment, threat, harm, death); this disconnection "extinguishes" the fear response. This is thought to result in adaptive responses to threatening situations in real-life events. Further, this theory suggests that nightmares are a failure of extinction, as the emotion is too great to process, and the fear response persists.

Adrenalin (in the form of norepinephrine) is present in our nervous systems during wakefulness, but less so in non-REM sleep, and basically absent in REM sleep. One theory of the disturbing dreams in patients with PTSD (post-traumatic stress disorder) is that the stress that initiated that disorder (characteristically, fierce combat experiences) is so severe as to trigger an outflow of adrenalin even in REM sleep, recurring as severe nightmares involving the patient's individual stressors, as flashbacks.

It is thought that medications that block adrenalin—and are used as such to treat high blood pressure—can help patients with PTSD; if adrenalin "overload" is prevented, a more normal extinction response to the fearful stimulus can occur, the emotional content of the nightmare may be lessened, and PTSD symptoms may improve. Clinical experience with this is mixed; some studies have shown improvement, some not.

What are we to make of the theories of dreams? We know that processing of memories (strengthening and weakening) occurs during sleep, and these memories may be reprocessed during dreams, perhaps sorting them further. Waking responses to negative emotions may be improved by dreams in the process of extinction. It is tempting to be pessimistic that progress in dream research may have limited results in the future, but it is reassuring to consider that newer brain-and neuron-function imaging techniques (such as fMRI and voltage emitting dyes) have already opened up new avenues of research into dreams; undoubtedly there will be newer, more revealing methods of dream analysis in the future.

In the last few decades, the concept of *lucid dreaming* has emerged. This means that one can learn to apply consciousness to dreams, to have wakeful-like consciousness during dreaming and be "consciously aware" that one is asleep and dreaming, even to interact during a dream. This seems like a contradiction in terms, in that one would be simultaneously conscious and unconscious, if we define sleep by that latter term.

We will discuss sleepwalking in a future chapter, but it helps to know that parts of the sleepwalking brain can be considered "asleep" (showing slow-wave N3 sleep) while other parts of the brain suggest wakefulness (the motor parts that control the physical aspects of sleepwalking, for example). EEG studies in lucid dreaming have not shown as precise a pattern, though.

Lucid dreaming is a technique that is helpful in chronic nightmare situations, as the sleeper can actively remind herself that she is, in fact, dreaming when that monster attacks, and even thwart the attack with preplanned activity in the dream, and ultimately decrease the frequency and severity of nightmares.

A more pleasurable application of lucid dreaming is the ability to direct one's own behavior in a dream with activities not available to us in the real world, like flying. Lucid dreaming takes practice and consistent effort to learn, easier for some than others. It shows promise in future dream research.[45]

CHAPTER 3

Some Answers

Running on empty

There are lots of ways *not* to sleep. No surprise there. The most common form of sleep deprivation is from behavioral habit: staying up too late for work, sex, exercise or entertainment; getting up too early for similar reasons, running around with a sleep deficit, a sleep "debt" owed to the brain to be paid back later, if at all.

This may be happening a bit less than in previous years as the general public is better-informed and more sophisticated about the importance of good sleep these days, but we still have a long way to go.

Remember Thomas Edison's claim that sleep was a waste of time? The military used to designate sleep as a luxury to be denied in soldiers' training and on tour, something "real men" (and women) could do without under extreme circumstances. In combat now, that may still be the case, but only for so long; remember, eventually sleep deprivation takes its toll, and if one stays up long enough, sleep always wins.

The armed forces have learned that adequate sleep is important for alertness in tense, and particularly in boring situations, as well as for good judgment in all situations. Studies of military and commercial pilots' competence after prolonged sleep deprivation have led to regulations about minimal sleep times prior to flying; "micro-sleeps" during actual approaches on landing an aircraft have been documented in pilots denied adequate sleep, and would give us all the willies if we thought that was still happening. (These and other studies resulted in regulations mandating minimal rest times between flights for pilots since then, as well as mandated napping opportunities on the longest flights.)

Consider the concept of a sleep deficit. Let's postulate that each of us has an optimal number of hours of sleep, an individual amount tagged to our particular brain function, that makes us feel the best each morning: we wake refreshed, we have good judgment and mood and alertness and cognitive ability every day until bedtime.

Remember the sleep deprivation studies in the previous section? Let's set up such a situation for our patient, Jake, a 39-year-old accountant, who usually gets eight hours of sleep nightly to be at his best, and he's doing it: getting about eight hours' sleep a night, doing well, going to bed at 11pm and getting up at 7am daily. That's 56 hours a week of good sleep, with 40 hours a week on weeknights and 16 on weekends.

Now let's inject a change: a new job or a new commute or a new gym routine, or a new girlfriend or a new baby. Something enters the picture to change his sleep habits. He now gets up an hour earlier, at 6am instead of 7am, and goes to bed half an hour later, at 11:30pm instead of 11. He's now averaging 6.5 hours of sleep a night, which comes to 32.5 hours a week during weeknights. If he starts this habit on a Sunday night we can say that he's 1.5 hours in "sleep debt" (a 1.5-hour sleep deficit) after one night, on Monday morning, and by Friday morning he's 7.5 hours in debt. (I'm using Sunday night through Thursday night as the "weeknights," as these are the most common nights before work or school.)

Now it's Friday evening, and our sleep-deprived Jake feels the 7.5 hours of sleep he has lost over the previous five days: he's tired at 4pm, he's grouchy, and he has a scraped tire on parallel parking from his "psychomotor" clumsiness, a problem he usually doesn't have. He is savvy enough to know he's behind on sleep, so his normal reaction is to say, "Okay, I'm just behind on sleep. I can make it up this weekend."

But *can* he? We suspect from our previous discussion that he can't. If he goes to bed on Friday and Saturday nights at 10pm and gets up at

8am Saturday and Sunday morning, he has achieved 10 hours of sleep each night, two hours more than usual, and has paid back his sleep debt with four hours of bonus sleep. Great. But he was *7.5 hours behind*, so he is nowhere near zero on the sleep balance sheet. And now Sunday night is here, and he reverts to his previous 11:30pm-to-6am sleep period, so his debt continues to mount.

If he does this for a few weeks or months, his new judgment-mood-alertness-cognitive-motor status becomes his "new-normal." He may not be aware of the changes (he may have become accommodated to it, as in the studies we discussed) or may assume they are normal reactions to a more intense work life or social life or exercise life. And they are, but from a sleep medicine point of view, they are pathologic: they are abnormal responses, potentially harmful to him, though in this instance reversible or avoidable. More sleep is the answer to a sleep debt, whether short- or long-term.

Here is the rule about short sleep: you can't make up for it on the weekends! The math above shows that. And even if you tried to make the numbers perfect (say, for example, Jake achieves an extra 7.5 hours of sleep every weekend, bringing his sleep debt to zero by Sunday morning), that doesn't undo the cycling that is occurring, with progressively more deficit all day each Monday through Friday, more mood and cognition problems, as the debt increases. It's as if *the brain charges interest and penalties* for sleep debt, so you can't pay it back hour-for-hour days later—*you must pay the debt every night*. In Jake's case, he has to get eight hours a night to feel perfect.

Do any of us do that? Do any of us get the perfect amount of sleep nightly? Not many, I think. We know there are lots of people who are truly sleep-deprived (less than seven hours of sleep a night chronically), but most of us hedge our sleep numbers from time to time. We just live with the consequences. In the sleep deprivation study we discussed earlier (see page 80), the researchers noted that the subjects tested as less sleepy after their recovery nights than they did *at baseline*, that is, less than when they entered the study.

The study was designed to filter out all but the most normal subjects for study, but inadvertently they found that these "normal" subjects were relatively sleep-deprived in their outside lives compared to when they were told just to get more sleep. They came to the study as "normal" but were in fact subtly sleep deprived, and being forced in the recovery part of the study to get normal sleep amounts made them report feeling better than when they started. This is one more piece of evidence that insufficient sleep is very common in the developed world.

For those who work during the daylight hours, a healthy number of nightly sleep hours is, hopefully, an achievable goal. But there are thousands of us whose work hours prevent normal, nocturnal sleep: those who work shifts, those who work nights, and those who work "rotating" shifts. With shift work, it's easy to see that evening shift work (working, say, from 3pm to 11pm daily) would be less disruptive than working night shift (11pm to 7am, for example).

One could get some semblance of a normal sleep period after working an evening shift: depending on the commute, one might get home and to bed by midnight and sleep until 8am. Unfortunately, late meals and housework sometimes get in the way. "Night owls" (those whose circadian rhythms (CRs) prompt late bedtimes and late risings) do better on evening shifts than "morning larks," whose CRs prefer early bedtimes and risings.

More on these groupings later.

A few people prefer night shifts, but most people do poorly working all night, and trying to sleep during the day. This behavior causes "circadian desynchrony," meaning the circadian rhythm cannot adapt to such a large change, and the brain is constantly fighting it. We teach night-shift workers to avoid bright light on the way home (to prevent more alertness which would prevent daytime sleep), to go to sleep soon after arrival home, with a dark bedroom with blackout curtains, a turned-off phone and a note on the doorbell to prevent interruptions.

But daytime sleep for night workers remains a problem, as it goes against our natural circadian rhythms, and many struggle to get even seven good hours of daytime sleep. This group is certainly at risk for mood/judgment/alertness/cognition problems. The time zone most at risk for them, the time when inadvertent sleep may cause a grave error, is around 3-6am, when sleep is not available to night shift workers... though inadvertent (and not so inadvertent) naps during nighttime work are common in this group.

Now a little personal history, just to illustrate how things have changed. When I was in training in the 1970s, in an Internal Medicine residency, our on-call rotation was called "every third." Here's what that meant: If I were "on-call" on a Monday, say, I would typically rise at 5:30am Monday morning, grab coffee and a shower, and get to the hospital at 6am. I would begin a pattern of patient chart reviews, inpatient hospital rounds with interns (for 20 to 30 patients), meetings with the teaching physicians, more rounds, calls to the Emergency Room to admit new patients, and perhaps a lecture in the afternoons, and maybe even a cardiac arrest or other disaster on the floors.

My usual day would be over at 6pm, but not on this night, as I'm the MD on call. That means I would stay at the hospital, and start taking calls from the other residents who were going home and signing out their patients to me. Once they had left, I was responsible for 60 to 80 patients, theirs and mine, for the next 12 hours. Nurses would call with problems that could be handled sometimes by phone, sometimes in person, throughout the night until 6am Tuesday when those residents returned and took over on their wards.

I might get 1–2 hours of sleep during the night, punctuated by more calls. From 6am until 6pm on Tuesday, the work pattern was the same as on Monday, until I signed out my patients to the new on-call MD before I could go home—having been at the hospital and mostly awake for *36 hours*. I could sleep Tuesday night at home, work a normal 6am–6pm day on Wednesday and sleep again, but then repeat the long work day/night on-call on the third day, Thursday. Weekends were the same.

Having almost no sleep over a 36-hour period was not then, and is not now, normal. It is also clearly not safe. Driving home after such sleep deprivation was risky: we now consider that to be "driving while impaired," but in the 1970s it was just part of the job. Once while driving home after having worked 36 hours, at around 6:30pm, I made a left turn *across the path of a stopped police car* at an intersection. When he pulled me over, I had no idea I had done anything wrong. It was not the only time police recognized my driving being impaired due to sleep deprivation, but luckily I never caused an accident.

Things have changed since the 1970s, mostly for the better. Even before the emergence of sleep medicine as a specialty and the explosion in research and knowledge about sleep and sleep deprivation, the law moved in to change the training experiences of all future medical students and trainees. The effects were dramatic.

In 1984, an 18-year-old named Libby Zion[46] died in a New York hospital from what later was judged to be a missed diagnosis: a treatable drug reaction, the error of which was blamed on lack of sleep of the treating physicians. Multiple lawsuits were filed against two medical residents who cared for her in the middle of the night as part of their 36-hour workday. Libby's father was a lawyer and a New York Daily News writer, and he later wrote "You don't need kindergarten to know that a resident working a 36-hour shift is in no condition to make any kind of judgment call—forget about life-and-death." As a result, laws were passed to limit on-call hours of trainees to no more than 24 hours at a time, and no more than 80 hours a week.

The change in laws helped. But since then, in the grand scheme of things, the problem of "working when you should be asleep" has not, and will not, go away. Private doctors are still woken up at night for medical problems, frequently have to drive to the hospital to see a patient in the middle of the night, and still get up to go to work for a full day the next day. Some doctors now have changed to working only night shifts in hospitals so others can sleep nights and workdays. Nurses work all shifts, as they have for years, as do firemen, policemen, first-responders, Amazon warehouse workers, and lots of others. All struggle with trying to cram the minimum needed amounts of sleep into the daylight hours of a given week, and all suffer the short-term and sometimes long-term problems of insufficient sleep.

In primitive societies, it may be possible for everyone to sleep at night and work all day (assuming no outside groups are threatening attacks requiring all-night sentries), but for the rest of the civilized world, we are stuck with the need for many people to give up their nocturnal sleep for the common good. It's a price we (actually, they, the night workers) pay. Be thankful if you're not one of those.

A person could develop a cold

Recall the 36-hour work shifts in the previous section? I fondly (well, TBH, not so much) remember those times and how I reacted to that degree of sleep deprivation: I routinely got a "cold" in the days following a bad night, with sniffles and fatigue (but usually not sore throat or cough or fever, so not that bad). Some but not all of my fellow residents reported the same response to on-call nights. It didn't take reading a lot of sleep research to realize that sleep deprivation somehow lowers our defense mechanisms.

We take it for granted that when we have an illness like a bad cold or the flu, that we will "take to our bed." We feel tired; we feel sleepy; we feel fatigued; we feel *awful.* Being vertical is a lot less attractive than lying down. It turns out that, in this as in most illnesses, there are dozens of chemical mediators of what comprises the "inflammatory response," which is the pattern of how we react to inflammation, as caused by infection or trauma. This response involves "sickness behavior," such as fever, chills, and loss of appetite, but also: *sleepiness.*

In the main, we think of the inflammatory response as a *healing* response: it represents mobilization of the body's resources to counter and reverse the damage caused by a pathogen or trauma. But it contributes to our "malaise" (feelings of illness) and sometimes causes further tissue damage when out of control.

Although it may seem logical to get sleepy when we're sick and to go to bed to save all our energy for healing, the interaction between sleep and illness is a bit more complicated—and interesting.

The mediators of the response to inflammation include proteins called *cytokines,* some of which promote further inflammation—are pro-inflammatory; and others are anti-inflammatory. I will try to simplify this discussion by homing in on just two of the many important cytokines that are pro-inflammatory: *interleukin-1* (IL-1) and *tumor necrosis factor* (TNF). These two play important roles in what we will see is a bidirectional relationship between sleep and inflammation.

Infections alter sleep. Viruses have been shown to affect sleep in animals and humans, including influenza, HIV, rabies, and rhinoviruses (responsible for colds). All viruses induce the production of IL-1 and TNF (and other cytokines) to promote the inflammatory response, which in most situations results in more total sleep—and this sleep consists of more than usual amounts of deep (N3) sleep, and less REM sleep. Bacterial infections (for example, from *Staph* or *E. coli*) similarly induce an inflammatory response that results in more deep sleep—along with all the other bad things that come from bacterial infections.

A dramatic example of how our proinflammatory friends affect sleep is in experiments where IL-1 and TNF are "painted" (coated) onto the cortex of only one side of a rat's brain; the result is sleep with slower brain waves (delta activity, or deep sleep) on the painted side, but not the unpainted side, of the brain. Inflammation promotes sleep, even regionally.

Coming in the other direction, consider the discovery that sleep deprivation promotes bacterial movement across the intestinal wall. Normally our "microbiome," that population of hundreds of different species of bacteria that colonize our intestine and make digestion (and many other facets of our health) possible, stays safely inside the intestines.

But sleep deprivation weakens the intestinal wall barrier, allowing so-called friendly bacteria to traverse the wall and enter the outside lymph channels where they are no longer friendly, where they don't belong, causing an inflammatory response—which promotes feeling ill, and sleepiness. So, sleep deprivation by this mechanism causes: sleepiness![47]

But if a night of sleep deprivation makes one feel ill, is this due to a real infection? Were my "cold" symptoms after a long night on-call due to an actual viral infection? Possibly not. Research has failed to show that short-term sleep deprivation worsens infection in rats or rabbits challenged with bacteria or viruses; we do not have similar challenge experiments in humans. (Long-term total sleep deprivation kills rats, but not humans.)

It appears more likely from all we know that the inflammatory response to sleep deprivation, with release of pro-inflammatory IL-1 and TNF, is responsible for those "cold" symptoms, not an actual infection. On the other hand, clinical insomnia, which is a form of chronic, partial sleep deprivation, is associated with more self-reported colds and even pneumonia in those sleeping less than five hours a night.

How does this all fit together? We can see how sleep deprivation, through the inflammatory response with IL-1 and TNF, causes inflammation, and inflammation causes sleepiness: this is a bidirectional relationship. The inflammatory response also causes malaise (feeling ill) that can mimic colds. Short-term sleep deprivation (a few nights) produces inflammation but not actual infection; long-term sleep deprivation in humans (months or more) may be associated with more respiratory infections.

If sleep loss and inflammation go hand in hand, it is not surprising that sleep problems (both fatigue and insomnia) are common in persons with inflammatory diseases, such as inflammatory bowel disease, lupus, and rheumatoid arthritis. When medications that specifically block TNF ("anti-TNF drugs") are given for some of these, sleep may improve, *even before the main symptoms of the disease (such as joint pain) improve*. This supports the idea that reducing inflammation improves sleep.

Think of insomnia now as a form of sleep deprivation. In keeping with the bidirectional concept, primary insomnia (insomnia not associated with any other illness) is associated with elevated cellular levels of IL-1 and TNF. An inflammatory marker commonly measured in blood tests is called *C-reactive protein* (CRP); in inflammatory situations, CRP levels rise along with IL-1 and TNF. CRP levels have been shown to be elevated in some patients with primary insomnia and to improve with treatment, one more connection between sleep loss and inflammation.

Consider treatment for insomnia. In America, drug therapy for insomnia is no longer considered "first-line therapy," given the potential side-effects and efficacy problems with sleeping pills. (We will address these problems in some detail later.) First-line therapy now is *cognitive behavioral therapy for insomnia*, known as CBTi, which works very well in most cases. The remarkable thing here is that CBTi, which is a form of "talk therapy," a non-chemical approach to a potentially inflammatory problem, has been shown not only to help insomnia—but to improve the associated inflammatory markers of it: our friends IL-1, TNF, and CRP.[48]

Again, the bidirectional relationship between sleep amounts and inflammation is evident. We can say that sleep itself is anti-inflammatory, and sleep loss is pro-inflammatory; good sleep improves levels of inflammatory markers, and sleep loss worsens them. As well, inflammation is anti-sleep, and anti-inflammation is pro-sleep: inflammation disrupts sleep patterns, promotes delta sleep and inhibits REM sleep; anti-inflammatories tend to normalize sleep quality. This has important implications in long-term sleep insufficiency situations, such as sleep apnea, insomnia, circadian rhythm disorders, pain syndromes, and many others, which by implication are problems with sleep quantity and quality that can then become problems with chronic inflammation.

Chronic systemic inflammation is considered a risk factor for heart disease, diabetes, and cancer. A recent model for chronic inflammation resulting in elevated risks for these outcomes is periodontal (gum) disease.[49] We will see in later chapters that sleep apnea, for example, is associated with higher risks of hypertension, diabetes, heart disease, and even cancer, and can speculate that the inflammatory component of the sleep loss that occurs chronically in sleep apnea may contribute to these risks.

The thief of dreams

Insomnia is another way we don't sleep. I will talk about this in more detail in Chapter Five, but suffice it to say here this is the most common sleep disorder in the developed world. Everyone has difficulty sleeping at one time or another, and as many as 40% of us consider ourselves to have a real problem with insomnia. There are formal definitions (of course): short-term insomnia is difficulty sleeping for less than three nights a week for less than three months, and chronic is more than three nights a week for more than three months. Insomnia can be classified as "sleep initiation insomnia," which is difficulty falling asleep, "sleep maintenance insomnia," which is difficulty staying asleep, and "mixed insomnia," which is both.

Studies have suggested that around 40% of patients complaining of insomnia have an underlying element of a psychological condition, anxiety or depression. This is not surprising, as we all know that anything that really bothers us psychologically can give us problems with sleep. Where this gets hairy is in chronic insomnia, when, after months of poor sleep, a person becomes so focused on nightly issues with getting to sleep that they develop "performance anxiety" in their degree of worry about being able to fall asleep... so they can't. A real, bidirectional, chicken-egg phenomenon. Sometimes both the anxiety and the primary or secondary insomnia must be dealt with simultaneously. Depression muddies this water even more.

What about those without anxiety? Insomnia can come from medications, but more commonly from overindulgence in caffeine and caffeine-like stimulants in coffee, tea, and even chocolate(!). Our tolerance to caffeine changes as we age so we may develop problems with it over time even if our "dose"—how much coffee we drink daily, for example— has not changed. Caffeine (remember that adenosine-blocker?) sneaks into soft drinks and dietary supplements and energy drinks and pre-scription medicines, and even cosmetics.

Coca-Cola has about a third as much caffeine (34 mg) as a cup of coffee (100–140 mg, depending on the cup size and brew strength, and Diet Coke more (46 mg), and energy drinks even more. Cold medicines and migraine medicines contain caffeine. Some skin creams can contain caffeine. Any quest to understand the cause of insomnia includes a search for intake of stimulants, especially caffeine. Intake can be obvious, such as in coffee or tea, or "occult," meaning hidden in foods or drinks or pills, such as diet drinks or cold medications. All can affect sleep, sometimes dramatically.

Situational insomnia may be short-term, or may morph into longer-term insomnia. We think of insomnia as having *predisposing, precipitating, and perpetuating factors.* Consider Maureen, a 37-year-old public affairs administrator, who has a family history of insomnia (mother and grandmother), but has never had the problem herself. This family history, this genetic inheritance, is her "predisposing factor."

Now let's say she has an unusual but serious misunderstanding with her employer, who accuses her of mismanaging a client, and she fears she will lose her job. This becomes the precipitating event for her, the external incident that triggers her genetic predisposition. She develops difficulty sleeping, in the form of early morning awakenings. She falls asleep normally, but wakes daily at 3–4am, frequently with thoughts racing through her mind about her work issue, and is further stressed that she can get no more than six hours of sleep nightly. She feels ragged most days after short sleep.

Then after six weeks of ongoing conflict at work, six weeks of anxiety and poor sleep, Maureen and her boss discover that the conflict was based on a reporting error, not her fault; she is absolved of all blame, and is back in the full graces of her employer, who apologizes and actually gives her a raise. She feels better during the day (about her job) and at night, but she is surprised to find that her insomnia persists, as bad as ever.

She still has early morning awakenings, and fights to go back to sleep every time. This is the perpetuating aspect of insomnia. In some patients it seems to develop a life of its own: Maureen now has a "habit" of sleeping poorly and may need help to reverse that. The good news is that the shorter the time of a problem with insomnia, the easier it is to treat. Therapy (cognitive behavioral therapy, or CBTi) can help. More on that later.

Then there's forced sleep deprivation, as in the evil practice of torture. This is important because of the effects of sleep deprivation have been known to torturers for centuries: that forced sleep deprivation (from loud noise, music, light, or pain) causes mood changes (anxiety, depression, and panic, not to mention fear) and cognitive difficulties, even hallucinations as deprivation becomes severe, resulting in lowered mental defenses and lowered resistance to enemy questioning.

Such techniques in some form were most recently and infamously used in the Abu Ghraib prison by the CIA during the US war in Iraq. There is always the question of whether information obtained through torture is reliable or true. Another question is whether sleep deprivation can break down inhibitions and resistance to pressure from authorities enough to prevent willful misrepresentation of information. Apparently, sometimes not.

Why, why, why

Give me a theory about why we sleep, and I'll press you to explain how your theory makes sleep mandatory. The Big Question—why we sleep—is a considered "one of the biggest mysteries in neurobiology."[50]

At the beginning of this book I procrastinated in answering the Big Question, "Why do we sleep?" Now perhaps we can put together what we have discussed so far, all that's new in sleep science that we have learned over the past 70 years, and ask—do we have the answer (or the answers) now?

My response would be: Yes, somewhat. And that in itself is a huge step forward.

Let's think a bit more about The Question. Let's agree that the best answers we come up with should explain the following:

1. Why do we need to sleep, as opposed to just resting while awake?

2. Why are different sleep stages necessary?

3. Why does sleep vary so drastically between different stages of life?

4. Why must the brain be disconnected from our environment (that is, "go to sleep" or "go offline") to accomplish whatever sleep does for us?

In the 1990s and 2000s I gave lectures to both physicians and the public entitled: "Why We Sleep." At the end of each lecture I teasingly ended with a slide showing nothing but a large question mark, finishing the talk with "We just don't know." And we didn't—there was no getting around the fact that we just *could not* explain why sleep is necessary. But we have come a long way since then.

Now I think we have partial answers to this question.

Here we arrive at the Big Reveal.

Remember in the section on page 74: "Cleanliness is next to..." we talked about the discovery of the cleansing system of the brain, the glymphatic system. And in the section "Thanks for the memories," we discussed the multiple ways that memories in sleep are both strengthened and discarded. Here then are two big parts in my attempt to answer the question: Why do we sleep?

Memory (learning and unlearning) and **brain cleansing.**

What we have learned about acquisition of memories during wakefulness with subsequent data and storage management during sleep suggests a prime reason to justify our sleep behavior.

What we have learned about the physical changes in the brain during sleep that promote the cleaning or "washing out" of the brain cells also should qualify as a primary function of sleep.

Memories are acquired during wakefulness, not during sleep.* That's why "sleep-learning" in the old-fashioned sleeping-with-lecture-tapes-and-headphones concept never worked. But sleep seems to provide a unique opportunity *to strengthen* memories and learning (by replaying

---

* Yes, I admit, you can remember some dreams.

them multiple times, at high speed, for example), *to store* memories for long-term access, and *to select* which memories are more important and which are not, so the less-desired ones can be weakened and discarded.

We assume that this memory management requires such a large share of the brain's resources that the brain must be reserved just for this purpose. We must be made "unconscious" to do this: the advantages of consciousness must be sacrificed to allow enough of the brain to be available for these efforts.

If we recall the rat's "place neurons," mapped during a maze while awake and then retraced during sleep many times at high speed, it's apparent that those same neurons could not be used for this purpose if they also had to be available for access during wakefulness, so the brain must be taken "offline" to allow this process.

Does the memory/learning function of our sleep justify two very different modes of sleep—REM and non-REM? Though we have discussed a number of differences in the types of memories and the ways memories are processed in different sleep stages, it is not clear yet why separate stages are needed here. Much of the research that has been done with sleep stages has involved selectively waking sleeping subjects whenever they showed on EEG the stage being studied—for example, waking patients every time they go into REM to assess what REM restriction might cause.

The problem with this is, that as the night goes on, the need for REM sleep (*REM pressure*) increases, and this appears to disrupt the non-REM sleep that is also being studied. In other words, our confidence in some of the subtle differences between stages (such as learning) may not be as clearcut as we thought. We do see more validity in some data observed directly in a stage, such as memory consolidation associated with "ripples" in deep (slow-wave) sleep. It's not so easy to isolate one sleep stage from another in research.

Dream research suggests that REM sleep is useful for processing and modifying *emotional* memories. It seems advantageous to be able to rework emotions and to optimize future emotional responses for our long-term benefit. We can speculate, since REM has characteristics more like wakefulness (rapid brain waves, a more active, warm brain) than slow-wave sleep, that it is during REM sleep that taking care of complicated emotions (as opposed to "simple" encoding of memories) is best performed.

Here is another Big Reveal: Emotional modification is thought to be one of the main reasons we dream in REM. We are refining and restructuring our emotional status in dreams.

We can therefore try to justify the two main modes of sleep with what we know of memory and learning during deep sleep, and dreaming and emotions in REM sleep. This earns a "pretty good" rating for satisfactorily explaining why we need two modes of sleep, but it will require much more data in the future to confirm this. And there is no reason to think that there may not be *other* differences between the stages that we currently cannot imagine.

Does our concept of sleep and learning justify how sleep varies in the different stages of life? It is easier to understand the need for much more sleep in infancy (up to 16 hours a day), childhood, and adolescence compared to adulthood (eight hours a day), as the required amount of learning is so much greater in those early years. One could argue that those years are *nothing but learning*, so the long sleep times we see then actually reinforce our understanding of the interplay between sleep and learning.

This question gets a fairly confident answer. Now let's look at the cleansing nature of sleep with regard to meeting these criteria.

The 2013 discovery of the glymphatic system allowed us to visualize channels "opening up" around brain vessels during deep sleep and subsequent clearance of waste products from the brain. This discovery also had implications for our understanding of brain anatomy as well as brain disease, most importantly the mechanisms of dementia.

But important as this new information may be, it does not by itself easily justify needing both REM and non-REM sleep. It seems that *it is only in the non-REM stage N3 (deep sleep)* that this cleansing process takes place, but admittedly we need much more information to understand how specifically stage-related this process is.

We can theorize that the greater electrical activity, anatomical growth, and metabolism of the brain in late childhood and adolescence may necessitate more cleansing during that time, and therefore more deep sleep. As we did with memory and learning during sleep, we can accept to some degree the basic need for cleansing that sleep satisfies, and agree that this, if correct, justifies the higher deep sleep requirements seen in youth.

Does this process explain the need for the brain to be "offline" for it to occur? If we consider the changes in the glial cells during deep sleep—decreasing their size and thereby increasing the channels between them and the brain's vessels, allowing more CSF (spinal fluid) to flow in and out of the brain—we can theorize that this would not work during wakefulness. (We say that only because it seems reasonable—and because this type of cleansing during wakefulness has not been found existing in nature yet.) It makes sense that nerve cell function during wakefulness might be disrupted by fluid shifts around the cells, conceivably less a problem during slow-wave sleep.

But this is speculation.

Where does this leave us? With an answer, of sorts, to one of the biggest questions about biology that has faced mankind over the ages: Why do we sleep?

Because we need to take time "offline" to process the input we've experienced during recent and not-so-recent wakefulness;

Because we need to store memories for long-term retrieval and to discard those we deem less helpful;

Because we need to process the emotional content of these memories to allow our later wakeful responses to similar fearful stimuli to be more constructive to our well-being;

And because we need to cleanse the brain of unwanted metabolic (waste) products of nerve cell metabolism and other proteins, lipids, and small molecules, to promote proper brain function and—so important for our time—possibly decrease the risks of dementia.

Make no mistake about it: this is a major milestone in the science of sleep.

Although sleep comprises a third of our human existence on Earth, the reasons for it have eluded our understanding for thousands of years. Even though there are many ways our understanding of these reasons for sleep may (and will) change in the next few decades, it seems reasonable to say that *we sleep to learn* and *we sleep to maintain our brains*.

If you remember nothing else from this book than this, you will be more enlightened about sleep than just about *almost everyone else who has ever lived on this planet.*

Really.

PART 2

THINGS THAT GO WRONG WITH SLEEP

This part of the book deals with different sleep disorders, that is, diseases. There is a fair amount of detail, particularly in the most common ones (obstructive sleep apnea and insomnia). I find all these disorders fascinating (as I should!) but not all readers will. If you or a loved one has sleep apnea, you may be interested in all of the sleep apnea section; if not, you may want to read the first part and skip past the sections on CPAP and other treatments. It's my hope you will find that the other sections (such as those on narcolepsy and circadian rhythm disorders) both informative and enlightening, even if you do not experience one of those problems.

They all teach us more about what sleep is and could be.

INTRODUCTION

I will now ask you to board a time machine with me.

We are going back to 1965, to the fictional office of Dr. Willis Mitchell, a fictional internist in Columbus, Ohio. Dr. Mitchell, a kind, intelligent, well-trained, and hard-working physician, has been in practice for 20 years and cares for both adults and adolescents. He also works hard to keep up with all the current medical knowledge, through meetings and journals. We will look at a few clinical problems that Dr Mitchell is faced with, and how he deals with them. We will see how his solutions to these problems differ from how they might be dealt with in the current century.

While enacting this time machine comparison we would highlight differences in diagnostic and treatment conventions, whatever the actual disease—we do things very differently with every medical problem now in the 2020s than in the 1960s—I think we will see that sleep problems are considered dramatically differently now, because back then, *no one knew that most of these problems even existed.*

We will discuss each of these sleep problems in more detail a bit later. For now, let's meet our first patient:

Scenario #1

John, 55, and his wife Mary, 51, are seeing Dr Mitchell because of John's snoring.

Mary: "Dr. Mitchell, you've got to help us! John snores so loudly at night I can no longer stay in the bedroom, and I miss being with him. And when we travel, it's impossible for me to sleep in the same hotel room with him. I have trouble controlling my anger at him, but I know it's really not his fault."

John: "I'm sorry to say this, Dr. Mitchell, but I'm not convinced I snore at all. I never hear that. But Mary, you do have occasional 'lady snores' too, and I don't complain about that."

Dr. Mitchell: "Snoring is common and usually is harmless. John, you may want to consider losing weight. I'm also going to send you to an ENT to see if there's a nasal cause. Otherwise, exercise and weight loss are the best suggestions I can make."

Unappreciated risk in 1965: Obstructive sleep apnea apnea (OSA). Medical risk level: Serious, even potentially fatal.

What would not have been addressed in 1965, as no one knew to ask, was whether Mary had noticed that John would snort, gasp, or otherwise stop breathing during sleep, and whether he was sleepy during the day. No one knew to connect John's known obesity, diabetes, high blood pressure, and (undiagnosed) coronary artery disease with his snoring into a single disease with its complications.

John would go on to fail in multiple attempts at weight loss, to have a negative ENT evaluation, to continue to snore, much to his wife's distress, and to leave her a widow six years later by dying of a heart attack at age 61. If you guessed that he had underlying obstructive sleep apnea, unheard of in 1965, with higher risks of high blood pressure, diabetes, heart disease, and early death, you would be correct.

Scenario #2

Marcus, 20, and his mother, Marcia, are seeing Dr. Mitchell because of Marcus' poor performance in school. Marcus lives at home and is a sophomore at a community college.

Marcia: "Dr. Mitchell, I'm desperate. Marcus is failing most of his classes even though he studies hard at night. In fact, I can't get him to go to bed as he studies so late! His teachers say he falls asleep in classes, but I don't see any sleepiness on weekends. He sleeps pretty late on weekends, though."

Marcus: "I just don't feel like sleeping when Mom thinks I should go to bed. I need to study because my grades are so bad, and I'm worried I might fail out of college."

Dr. Mitchell: "Marcus, I just want to make sure you're getting up early enough so you'll be sleepy at night. No more sleeping late! And I'm going to ask you to cut back on the soft drinks, which have caffeine in them."

Unappreciated risk in 1965: Delayed sleep phase syndrome (DSPS). Medical risk level: Moderate to severe

What would not have been addressed in 1965 would be Marcus' overall pattern of sleep and wake. Since puberty he had involuntarily gone to bed later and later (as late as 2–3am) and awakened each morning later and later (as late as 12–1pm). On school days he struggled to get up early (at 7am) but then fell asleep in his morning classes. On weekends, if he slept late, he felt completely normal and alert all day. The problem was not that he needed to get up earlier, but that his sleep phase had shifted to be abnormally late. This disorder, called delayed sleep phase syndrome, was unheard of in 1965 but is now easily treatable (with melatonin and light) once diagnosed.

Scenario #3

Frank, 55, an accountant, and his wife Carla, are seeing Dr. Mitchell for his kicking during sleep.

Carla: "You have to help us, Dr. Mitchell! Frank's is kicking his legs all night and I can't sleep. He doesn't really hurt me but I try to stay away from him in bed. That's hard to do as we sleep in a double. Some nights he doesn't kick at all. When he does kick, the kicks come every 20 seconds! I've even timed them."

Frank: "I know this is a problem for her, Dr. Mitchell, but it doesn't bother me at all. I sleep fine, but the sheets are sometimes all awry when I wake up."

Dr. Mitchell: "Your exam is normal. I'm going to do an X-ray of your hips and legs to see if anything's there. Are you sure you're not just anxious from problems at home or work?"

Unappreciated risk in 1965: Periodic limb movement disorder. Medical risk level: Mild to moderate.

What would have gone unexplained in 1965 is now called *periodic limb movements* (PLMs), a disorder previously thought part of a bigger problem called *restless legs syndrome*. PLMs are quite common and can bother people a lot, but usually only the bedpartner, not so much the sleeper. It may not have any long-term health effects. Dr. Mitchell has no way of knowing what it is, or what treatment to suggest.

Scenario #4

Leo, 64, a lawyer, and his wife, Miriam, 59, are seeing Dr. Mitchell for his nightmares.

Miriam: "Dr. Mitchell, I am so worried about Leo. Every week or so he has a nightmare and begins yelling in his sleep, sometimes even kicking and punching. I can't wake him even when I yell back. See this bruise on my cheek? He hit me! But I know he didn't mean it— he was so apologetic after! What can we do?"

Leo: "I feel terrible about this, Dr. Mitchell. I tell myself it won't happen again, but then it does. I´m usually dreaming I'm being attacked by some guy or some animal, and I have to fight my way out. Next thing I know I wake up with her yelling at me and I'm on the floor. I just can't go on hurting Miriam like this."

Dr. Mitchell: "I am going to adjust your diet and take you off all alcohol. I want to make sure you're getting enough sleep and maybe a vacation from work would help. I am also going to refer you for marriage counseling in case there is some underlying tension between the two of you prompting this kind of behavior."

Unappreciated risk in 1965: REM sleep behavior disorder. Medical risk level: Moderate to severe

What could not be discussed in 1965, because no one had yet described it, was a disorder now called *REM sleep behavior disorder* (RBD). Unfortunately, none of the treatments Dr. Mitchell recommended was helpful for this. Leo's nightmares would go on to get worse and eventually he and Miriam would have permanently separate bedrooms, and Leo's rapid deterioration from Parkinson's disease and dementia starting at age 65 and his death at the age of 68 are blamed in part on RBD—or would have been, had it been understood then.

What do all these scenarios have in common? They all describe sleep disorders that were prevalent in 1965—lots of people had them; many suffered from them, and some died from them—but back then no one knew that these problems even existed. No doctors knew how to diagnose or treat them. Even though REM sleep was discovered in the 1950s, the explosion in research in sleep science began in the 1970s, which has exponentially increased since then. Likewise, knowledge about sleep disorders—what they are, how to treat them—has become increasingly available over the last 50 years.

This is, of course, the essence of the second part of this book.

Let's now turn to obstructive sleep apnea (OSA), which is unique in the following way. For centuries it has affected a large part of the population (up to 25% of middle-aged men[51] now, for example) and caused significant disability (disabling daytime sleepiness, fall-asleep accidents, hypertension, diabetes, heart attacks, strokes, atrial fibrillation, and death)—but before the 1960s, *no one even knew the disease existed.* No one knew there was a problem. It was hiding in plain sight.

When patients suffered and died from OSA, the problems were always attributed to something else. Of course, there are numerous diseases that have been known for centuries but misunderstood until recently—such as congestive heart failure, malaria, and diabetes—but these were recognized as problems to be solved, and various (usually worthless) treatments were tried. Physicians could see that something was wrong though they did not understand the pathology required to come up with effective treatment.

In the case of sleep apnea, in contrast, no one even suspected that there was a disease there *at all.*

Now we are treating patients by the thousands with this problem, and their health is all the better for it. Other diseases that have been "discovered" in recent years, such as anomalous coronary artery disease—when a coronary vessel has grown into the wrong place and can cause cardiac arrest in young people—may be examples of diseases that have been around forever, have dramatic implications for health, and have avoided detection for centuries—but these diseases affect only a small percentage of the population.

Sleep apnea is very common, can be very severe, and has been around for centuries. These days one would be hard pressed to find someone who doesn't know someone, or at least know of someone with sleep apnea, or even have sleep apnea themselves.

In this sense, there has never been a disease like sleep apnea before.

CHAPTER 4

Too sleepy*

Obstructive sleep apnea

This is a disease that spawned an international medical specialty. The prevalence and frequency of sleep apnea as a clinical disease brought sleep medicine out of the obscure world of research and into the much wider and visible clinical arena. This resulted in recognition of sleep medicine as a clinical specialty and eventually sleep medicine's achievement of "board" status: to have its testing criteria for clinical competence recognized by the American Board of Medical Specialties. Without the distinction of "board certification," one cannot tell a trained from a non-trained specialist, so this achievement was key to academic as well as public recognition and acceptance of sleep medicine.

Because of its high prevalence in the community, sleep apnea has spawned the emergence of thousands of sleep laboratories around the

---

* When I began studying sleep disorders in the 1990s, we simplistically divided sleep problems into three groups. These were called DOES, DIMS, and others. DOES stands for "disorders of excessive sleepiness," and DIMS for "disorders of initiating and maintaining sleep;" "others" is everything else. These abbreviations are not used much anymore because the distinctions were not precise enough, but for our purposes they make a handy way to think of these problems. Not all the patients with sleep apnea, for example, are sleepy, but because sleepiness is an important consideration in all such patients, we still think of OSA as an example of "DOES."

world. Had it not been for such a high demand for diagnosis of sleep apnea, only universities and research facilities would have been able to justify the labor- and cost-intensive efforts it takes to maintain a sleep laboratory, and many of the other sleep disorders we will be discussing would have been much harder to understand and diagnose. There are now accredited sleep laboratories in every large and almost every medium-sized city in the USA; this has contributed to the explosion in knowledge of sleep disorders from which we all benefit, and that prompted the writing of this book.

The word "apnea" means "not breathing" (specifically, "no flow"), and obstructive apnea means this is happening because of a blockage somewhere. When that happens during sleep, we get obstructive sleep apnea, or **OSA**. (We also recognize *central sleep apnea*, a different, less common disorder we will discuss separately. But here when we use the shorthand phrase "sleep apnea," we are referring to the *obstructive* type of apnea, or OSA.)

Obstructive sleep apnea comes in three major flavors: tonsillar-based, tongue-based, and soft-palate-based. These are the areas that can "crowd" the back of the throat, usually causing no problem during wakefulness, but during tissue relaxation, during sleep, may proceed from just crowding to complete obstruction. Other areas, like the lateral (side-) walls of the throat can contribute to the crowding, as can the back wall of the throat. In children, the tonsillar version is most common and can sometimes be cured with tonsillectomy. In adults, the soft palate is most commonly the villain, especially in the obese, but the tongue is not far behind, and some adults have obstruction at both levels.

It gets more complicated when we consider the size and position of the jaw, as a small jaw or a jaw that does not extend out very far (resulting in a "weak chin" or an overbite) can position the tongue further back in the throat, making it more likely to obstruct during sleep. Sleep physicians assess these variables in a physical examination. Nasal obstruction seems to contribute to snoring but not so much to obstructive apnea—because apnea from nasal obstruction is easily overcome by opening and breathing through the mouth.

In men, OSA may emerge as early as puberty, when body changes and weight gain are rapid, and its frequency increases with age and with weight gain, becoming most apparent in middle age. Becoming overweight (body mass index, or BMI 25.0–29.9) and especially obese (BMI 30.0 or above) promotes OSA, but somewhere between a quarter and a third of all OSA patients are of normal or low weight. This is the group more likely to have their apnea caused by jaw (mandibular) issues that affect tongue position; there are plenty of thin people with sleep apnea (I happen to be one of them).

In adult women, the frequency of OSA is much less than in men from the time of puberty until menopause, when it increases dramatically, nearly equaling that in men. This is not explained by the difference in testosterone levels between men and women, but in part is related to weight gain that frequently occurs after menopause.

OSA is suspected whenever snoring, witnessed apneas, and daytime sleepiness occur. While snoring is almost universal, not everyone has witnessed apneas (because not everyone has a bedpartner, and not every bedpartner hears the pauses, snorts, and gasps that signal apneas during sleep), and only about 60% with true OSA have daytime sleepiness. The issue of sleepiness is important because not only do those with daytime sleepiness have more fall-asleep accidents and more cognitive and mood problems, but this group also has more hypertension, heart disease, and insulin resistance related to OSA.

Since its first description in the mid-20th century, OSA has been "graded" by counting the frequency of stopping breathing during sleep, as measured during a standard in-lab sleep study. Breathing stoppages have long been divided into complete or partial, but the partials have recently been further divided into more subtle versions.

A full cessation of flow (for a minimum of 10 seconds) constitutes an *apnea*. A partial cessation is counted if airflow drops below baseline and is associated with a drop in oxygen level or an arousal (brief awakening) from sleep. This is called a *hypopnea*. The most subtle abnormality is a flattening of the inspiratory curve in the breathing channel; when this is followed by an arousal, it is called a *RERA*, or respiratory effort-related arousal. The concept is that subtle narrowing of the throat limits the flow breathing in; this increased effort to breathe in eventually causes an arousal in the brain. Having lots of these arousals can cause more sleep disruption with resultant daytime sleepiness, plus other symptoms.

For decades the classic sleep score for OSA was called the "apnea-hypopnea index," or AHI. This was derived by counting all the apneas and hypopneas over the whole night and dividing that number by the number of hours of sleep. As more significance has been attributed to the more subtle forms of breathing problems, we now more commonly use the "respiratory disturbance index," or RDI, which is apneas plus hypopneas plus RERAs, divided by the hours of sleep. OSA is now graded as follows:

Normal: RDI 0–5 events per hour
Mild: RDI 5–15 events per hour
Moderate: RDI 15–30 events per hour
Severe: RDI 30 or more events per hour

Sleepiness is measured as objective (measured by standardized test—the MSLT) or subjective (measured by questionnaire). You may recall from our discussion of the MSLT (page 59) that sleepiness is measured in the lab in the evaluation of narcolepsy or idiopathic hypersomnia, but is too expensive for more frequent use. Subjective sleepiness is measured most commonly with the Epworth Sleepiness Scale, or EES, developed by the Australian sleep physician Murray Johns in 1991.[52] The question-naire asks individuals to rate their likelihood of dozing in eight common situations, such as watching television or sitting quietly after lunch. Each situation is scored from 0 (would never doze) to 3 (high chance of doz-ing), producing a total score ranging from 0 to 24. Scores above 8-10 are generally considered suggestive of excessive daytime sleepiness. This questionnaire is so helpful (and short) that we ask every patient to fill it out on every visit to our sleep clinic to assess their sleepiness status and response to treatment. There are a number of other questionnaires used to assess sleepiness that are used more commonly in research.

Suppose I were to tell you that, unbeknownst to you, a malevolent troll sits outside your bedroom door each night and magically knows when you fall asleep. As soon as you do, he creeps in, wraps his evil little hands around your neck, and strangles you until you wake up. When you do, he lets go. You gasp and startle awake. He runs out of the room. You look around but see nothing wrong. You don't wake completely and don't know why you woke, nor remember being strangled. Most of the time you don't even remember awakening. But each time, as soon as you fall back asleep, he comes back in and does it again. And again. And again.

He is doing this, let's say, 200 times a night for every eight hours you sleep (he's very persistent) for the last few *years*. You might logically ask, "Is that why I feel so tired all the time? Because I'm being awakened 25 times every hour all night long? Every night for *years*?" The answer would be yes. Now if we could measure your breathing while the troll is at work on your neck, we might find that sometimes he throttles you so severely that you get no air in at all (an apnea, a complete cessation of breathing), but at other times during strangulation you wake before breathing completely stops, and he has to run out while you are still getting small amounts of air in (an hypopnea, a partial stoppage).

There are even times when the troll mischievously squeezes your throat so very slowly that you are forced to work harder and harder to get air in; you finally wake while he's still squeezing, so he lets go (this would be a RERA, a respiratory effort-related arousal). You awoke before a complete stoppage of breathing occurred, but your sleep still gets disrupted. The troll still runs out of the room when you wake. Annoying little troll!

This adds up to an RDI (200 apneas and hypopneas and RERAs divided by eight hours of sleep) of 25 events per hour, or moderate OSA.

What does snoring have to do with it? Snoring is the noisy vibrating of tissues in the back of a sleep-crowded throat (remember the soft palate? The tongue base? Can be either or both) which does indeed limit flow of air into your lungs but is not severe enough to cause an arousal nor a drop in oxygen levels. Snoring can be *very* noisy (there are anecdotal reports of patients suffering hearing loss from their own snoring), even getting up into the chainsaw-in-the-bedroom level (over 100 decibels).

Isn't it amazing that *any* marriages can survive snoring?

Speaking of marriages, now consider that your bedpartner is with you and the sleep physician when you're discussing that malignant troll that's strangling you every night. You're not surprised when your partner says, "So that's why I hear him gasping like that all night long! And that's why he's so drowsy all day. That's why he never seems to listen to me!"

Now imagine the stress you experience every time you are the victim of moderate OSA, which is the equivalent of repeated attempted murder. It makes sense that stress hormones, like norepinephrine (a form of adrenalin) surge in your bloodstream every time you're strangled, and your blood pressure and heart rate shoot up. In this case, that's 200 shots of adrenalin kicking at your heart and your blood vessels every night, or about 73,000 times a year. Seventy-three thousand jolts that normal sleepers never experience. Every year.

Perhaps that makes it less surprising to learn that OSA, especially if it is moderate or severe, may predispose to sustained high blood pressure, heart disease (heart attacks, congestive heart failure), abnormal heart rhythms (particularly atrial fibrillation), strokes, prediabetes (insulin resistance), type II diabetes, and early death. We know that weight gain can predispose to hypertension, diabetes, and heart disease, and now we can consider that OSA with obesity is one more risk factor for these complications.

Vascular damage is the risk inherent in high blood pressure, with trauma to the sensitive cells of the vessel walls occurring from the elevated pressure to which they are subjected. When OSA causes a large number of surges of pressure added to this already-high pressure, as well as increases in heart rate from surges of norepinephrine with each apnea, it's no surprise that more vascular damage occurs. Add to this the extra risks to the vessels from high cholesterol in many patients and, worse, the inflammatory component of obesity which adds to vascular damage (not to mention the inflammatory aspect of the associated sleep deprivation!), and one starts to wonder how any OSA patient can survive without treatment.

The connection between OSA and atrial fibrillation (and the optimism that OSA treatment helps atrial fibrillation in many ways) is now so well recognized that many patients with newly diagnosed atrial fibrillation are automatically referred for OSA screening. Many seemingly asymptomatic OSA patients are found this way.

Diabetes also contributes to vascular disease (diabetes seems to damage smaller vessels more than the larger ones), which explains the increased risks of stroke and heart attack in diabetics; the elevated risk of type II diabetes in OSA seems related to the severity and number of drops in oxygen level that occur in each night of OSA, rather than the mechanical or hormonal effects of the obstructions.

A useful rule of thumb in OSA with relation to hypertension and diabetes has to do with "dipping." Normally, our blood pressure and our blood sugar are both lower on awakening in the morning than on retiring at night. This makes sense—we are usually taking in neither food nor water all night, which promotes lower blood sugars and blood pressure in the mornings. But OSA patients are said to be "non-dippers," with blood pressures and blood sugars higher in the mornings, not dipping lower.

This makes sense given the surges in both blood pressure and blood sugar that patients with OSA experience all night long—especially if theirs is moderate to severe. This fact is occasionally helpful when patients wonder if they need screening for OSA and have the availability of a blood pressure cuff or blood sugar measurement at home (as long as they understand the test is not 100% sensitive). Finding a morning pressure or blood sugar higher than that at bedtime is a clue that OSA could be a problem. Home studies or full sleep studies may then be the next step.

Alcohol, even in low doses, can have profound effects on the severity of obstructive sleep apnea. It selectively relaxes the musculature of the upper airway, increasing airway collapsibility and leading to more snoring, longer and more frequent apneas, and greater drops in oxygen levels during sleep. Alcohol also blunts arousal responses, allowing breathing disturbances to persist longer before recovery occurs. In addition, regular alcohol use may contribute to weight gain, which can further worsen sleep apnea over time. For patients with obstructive sleep apnea, limiting or avoiding alcohol—especially in the evening—is one of the most effective steps toward reducing disease severity and lowering the risk of complications.

Excessive daytime sleepiness (EDS) is a risk for all patients with OSA; some complain of marked sleepiness, while others are unaffected. (It's frequently harder to persuade those who are not sleepy that they should consider treatment, as they feel relatively well.) EDS can be defined as a high Epworth Sleepiness Score (ESS, see page 132) greater than 10, but can also include those who are deathly sleepy all day or those who just drag around with fatigue or lassitude all day without a real impetus to fall asleep. EDS can be caused by sleep deprivation alone or by disorders that disrupt sleep like OSA and others we'll discuss later. When it is severe, EDS can be life-threatening: motor vehicle accidents, for example, are more common for drivers with OSA, especially in those who combine OSA with sleep deprivation.

Thomas, a 55-year-old 18-wheeler truck driver with undiagnosed OSA has to work extra shifts and night shifts to make ends meet. He is sedentary (sitting down driving eight or 12 or more hours a day) and, at 304 pounds, adds obesity as risk factor for OSA. He frequently works late hours and misses sleep, and lately has been driving all night to make important deliveries. Yesterday he had only six hours of sleep—from 5am to 11am, after an overnight drive—but during each six hours of sleep he was awakened 150 times by his moderate sleep apnea (with RDI 25, like you in the example above). He is unaware of this.

At 1pm yesterday he started a planned 16-hour drive, with only bathroom and truck-stop breaks. At 3am on a remote highway travelling at 70 mph in his tractor-trailer, his sleep deprivation (too little sleep) and his sleep apnea (poor quality sleep) from the*

---

* Because the risks of undiagnosed sleep apnea have been recognized, most states require drivers holding commercial drivers' licenses to be tested for OSA and even checked for compliance with therapy yearly. Also, restrictions on hours of continuous driving without intervening rest have been legislated.

day before join forces with his circadian drowsiness (high at 3am), and his eyes begin transiently, and then permanently, to close. Involuntary sleep takes over. He is so sleep-deprived that he jumps right into stage N2 sleep while still moving at 70 mph. All this is happening just as he comes over the top of a hill; what he doesn't see in front of him is a line of traffic stopped in both lanes.

He does not survive the subsequent impact, nor do three of the people in the 11 cars that are involved in the crash. Cars and people are strewn across the highway. The subsequent accident investigation notes that there are no skid or swerve marks leading up to the site of impact, indicating that there were no brakes applied nor steering efforts made to try to avoid a crash. No mechanical problems are found in what remains of the 18-wheeler. The investigation concludes that the cause of the accident was "driver fatigue."

This is characterized as a "single-vehicle accident" in the sense that the driver was asleep as he came over the top of the hill and was probably going to go off the road on his own had his truck not been impeded by a line of stopped cars. True single vehicle accidents—those who crash or drive off the road by themselves for no obvious reason—are usually attributed to "fatigue," which is DOT-speak for "probably asleep at the wheel." These accidents occur more between 1am and 7am and particularly between 1am and 4am, which fits with our understanding of circadian dips in alertness at night. Traffic reports do not contain information about underlying sleep disorders, so we have no way to know if many of these also involve undiagnosed OSA.

We can think of EDS in persons with OSA as an advanced form of sleep deprivation. Getting too little sleep is one thing, but getting too little sleep *that in itself* is poor quality sleep seems to worsen the issue. We know from Chapter Three that sleep loss causes problems with cognition, mood, judgment, and even motor function.

The "perfect storm" for an accident to happen, whether at the wheel of a car, the locomotive of a train, the helm of an oil tanker, the flight deck of an airliner, or the control panel of a nuclear power plant would be to have a critical operator in charge who is: (1) working at night on (2) insufficient sleep with (3) a background of untreated obstructive sleep apnea. And if big accidents can occur in this setting, just think how many smaller errors in calculation and judgment can occur this way in all occupations and social situations. It's something one could lose sleep just thinking about.

PEARLS OF WISDOM

Obstructive sleep apnea is very common but is undiagnosed in perhaps two-thirds of those who have it. If you have any of the signs or symptoms during sleep—snoring with gasping or snorting and/or unexplained daytime sleepiness—evaluation and treatment will likely improve and even prolong your life. Sleep studies are now easily done at home and are not expensive. In most cases, your primary care doctor will be able to refer you to a sleep physician to find out if you have it, and how severe it is.

Treatment of obstructive sleep apnea

The treatment of OSA sometimes produces dramatic improvement and, over the decades, has become progressively easier. When this problem was first recognized as upper airway blockage in the mid-20th century, the logical treatment was to bypass the obstruction, and the only way known to do this then was with tracheostomy: a surgical opening in the neck below the level of the throat. This allowed breathing to occur in and out through the hole during the night and permitted a more normal level of sleep. A plug could be placed in the hole during the day so that breathing and speaking could be performed normally. This procedure, although now (and even then) considered somewhat radical, undoubtedly saved lives.

You can imagine the resistance to tracheostomy in these early days for most people with this "sleep apnea" problem they had never heard of:

Physician: "Mr. Sanders, we have determined that you have sleep apnea, and the best treatment is a tracheostomy."
Mr. Sanders: "What?!! You want to put a permanent hole in my neck for snoring? Are you kidding me?"

Obviously, the physician knew that the surgery would be to cure more reasons than just snoring; the few medical experts dealing with this in the early days understood that sleep quality, oxygen levels, and daytime sleepiness could improve with tracheostomy, and that life expectancy itself was likely to improve. But in that time (the 1960s and 1970s), other complications we now associate with untreated OSA were not yet appreciated: hypertension, diabetes, heart disease, strokes, atrial fibrillation, motor vehicle accidents, and others. As so often happens with newly recognized diseases, the most severe cases are the easiest to identify and therefore are the first diagnosed and treated, and those in the mild and moderate categories go undiagnosed and untreated at first. This was certainly true with OSA in the beginning: the most severe cases merited treatment, especially since the treatment was so difficult, and the milder cases were not detected.

The breakthrough in treatment occurred in June 1980. Colin Sullivan, a pulmonologist and professor at the University of Sydney, New South Wales, Australia, had a patient with severe OSA who refused tracheostomy. Understanding the site of the obstruction in the throat, he reasoned that forcing air into the back of the throat might hold the tongue or soft palate away from the back wall of the throat, thus preventing obstruction to airflow. Using a stock vacuum cleaner, he reversed the airflow in the tubing by hooking it to the output of the machine, so it "blew" instead of "sucked." Applying this flow to the patient's face with a mask using "rapid-setting silicone sealant," he observed:

Within minutes of the full polysomnography setup, the patient had gone to sleep and developed repetitive severe sleep apnea. I gradually increased the air pressure in the circuit, and suddenly the apnea stopped and normal breathing appeared. It was an incredible result. As we watched in amazement, the patient went into REM sleep. I quickly decided to repeat the experiment by dropping the pressure, and the apnea recurred. I went through a series of cycles increasing the pressure and so literally "turning off" the apnea, and then dropping the pressure and "turning on" the apnea. There was no uncertainty or ambiguity. The method worked.

We decided to leave the patient on the pressure for the rest of the night. We watched as he continued to sleep for around seven hours, without any apnea, and with the most extraordinarily intense sleep patterns. The patient's response the next day was equally exciting. He was awake and alert for the first time in years.[53]

Dr Sullivan went on to develop the world's first dedicated treatment for sleep apnea, called Continuous Positive Airway Pressure, or CPAP. Over the next few decades, CPAP devices became (compared to a vacuum cleaner) smaller, quieter, easier to use, with lots of "bells and whistles" like humidifiers, sophisticated air pressure contours, and even self-adjusting options. Today something like eight million people sleep with CPAP in the USA, and millions more around the world, with dramatic effects in many cases.

One of the most rewarding aspects of sleep medicine is that "miracle" that OSA patients describe on their first visit back after starting CPAP: they are delighted, and their bedpartners are overjoyed; they no longer snore; they are awake all day; their mood and thinking and memory all seem better. I have spent this first CPAP visit with hundreds of patients, and, as a physician, it can certainly make one's day.

But not everyone has this experience. Some patients cannot tolerate CPAP from the outset, and overall, about 40% of all patients given CPAP stop using it after a few months. The reasons are many: pressure problems, mask fit problems, noise, dryness, tubing issues, and so on. But what stands out to me after working for years to help people with OSA adapt to CPAP is this: it is the quality of the *entire team* that is involved with the patient that sets the stage for success or failure with CPAP. This includes the sleep physician, the nurses, the CPAP distributing companies, and, most importantly, *the sleep technologists.*

The sleep techs (who deliver the machine, teach the patient and family how to use it, help choose and fit the mask) make the most difference in future success, and help with problems later. The sleep techs have the technical answers to all the questions that arise in the first few months of CPAP use, and that makes all the difference in patients´ compliance and thus quality of life.

In the early days of CPAP (the 1990s), the insurance companies decided that sleep techs were not necessary and money could be saved by direct delivery of the machine to the patient. We called this "drive-by CPAP," as the distributor would deliver a machine to a patient's home with little if any instruction or fitting, leaving the patient to figure it out on their own. Not surprisingly, the likelihood of success with CPAP for patients using it nightly afterwards plummeted. In fact, we found that once a patient became disillusioned with CPAP, it was difficult if not impossible to get them to try it again: we called this "poisoning the well."

The essence of a good experience with CPAP starts with the physician educating the patient on the severity and complications of their OSA, and the reasons for starting CPAP. The next step is the delivery of the machine, preferably in the medical office, with detailed explanation by the sleep tech as to how to use the machine and, most importantly, help with choosing and fitting the mask. Follow-up visits with the physician and with the techs in the future optimize the chances of success with CPAP.

Here we get into the nitty-gritty of the details of CPAP. There are literally hundreds of choices of masks on the market; no one mask design fits all faces. We are beginning to see artificial intelligence used for custom mask-fitting. CPAP machines generally all have the same pressure limits but there are lots of different ways of delivering the pressure (or pressures, in some cases), and the settings depend on the severity of the OSA.

Humidifiers on the machines can turn a bad experience into a good one. Tubing from the machine to the patient may have its own heating elements to prevent water condensation. And so on. But suffice it to say that the devil is in all of this detail; patient satisfaction depends entirely on whether they are handled well by the whole team. A fragmented team makes for a fragmented experience.

Almost all CPAP machines now are recording devices, allowing the team to follow usage details such as hours of use, pressures used, and even an estimate of residual abnormal breathing while on treatment. This allows the team to adjust pressures for improved comfort and elimination of OSA, and to advise patients on the need for more hours of use. These days the team can even download the data remotely to the medical office, while the patient's machine remains at home.

Do patients like CPAP? Some love their CPAPs, especially those who are very sleepy before treatment and who get a miraculous sense of alertness after treatment. It's gratifying to see someone so delighted with their result, so that any issue with the treatment device seems minor. Many OSA patients have little or no daytime sleepiness; they may be referred by their terrified bed partner, who fears they won't survive the night, or by a physician who links their hypertension or heart disease or atrial fibrillation with risk of OSA.

For reasons we don't yet understand, a majority of OSA patients with heart disease, atrial fibrillation, and/or strokes are in this non-sleepy category, even when their OSA is severe. This group can be harder to persuade to use CPAP nightly. They may feel minimally better or no better at all with diligent use of CPAP, so convincing them to continue may require a good team effort to explain that the complications of OSA are still serious risks, even though the patients feel fairly well.

The available statistics can be troublesome. Some, but not all, research supports the concept that CPAP usage lowers the risk of future heart attack, stroke, and death; some conclude that only CPAP usage more than four hours a night achieves those goals. The problem may be that, decades ago, Medicare defined "CPAP compliance"—*for funding purposes only*—as usage of more than four hours a night, but somehow this definition was later adopted into research to separate the "users" from the "non-users." If we think of CPAP as restoring "good sleep" and sleep without CPAP as "rotten sleep," and if we remember that insufficient sleep is less than six hours a night (see Chapter Two), then giving the CPAP seal of approval to those who achieve only four hours of "good sleep" with it makes no sense.

Think of it this way. You're trying to set up an experiment to prove or disprove that CPAP prevents heart attacks in people with sleep apnea. Each person's CPAP machine tells you how many hours per night they are using them. You want to create two groups for comparison: one group of "good users" and one of "poor users," expecting that the good users will get more benefits from CPAP, possibly fewer heart attacks.

But where do you draw the "usage" line between the two groups? Again, for all otherwise normal sleepers, we consider less than six hours a night as insufficient sleep, with all the complications (including heart problems) that entails. We believe that CPAP promotes "normal sleep," but only when the mask is on. So, wouldn't you want to divide your CPAP users into two groups that use their machines more, or less, than six hours?

Seven hours might be even better, since that's the recommended sleep amount for all normals (see page 54), so you might even have three groups, the "poor users" with less than six hours a night and the "good users" with more than seven hours, and a group you call "borderline users with between six and seven hours. Remember, for purposes of research we equate "CPAP sleep" with "normal sleep," so our time limits for each are the same.

Thus we would doubt the conclusions of a study (or group of studies)[54,55] that contends that CPAP does *not* prevent heart attacks in "good users," if a patient could be a "good user" by sleeping with CPAP just over four hours a night—because four hours of sleep is still insufficient, and itself promotes heart disease. Hard as it might be to achieve, a goal of *seven* hours of CPAP usage should be the gold standard for research, the cutoff for separating the users from the non-users.* I believe large studies using

---

* Seven hours of nightly use was the goal we set for all our CPAP users in the medical clinic; our motto was "All Night, Every Night," and we wore lapel buttons that said just that.

this criterion in research on OSA in heart disease patients would show stronger effects of CPAP in preventing future major acute cardiovascular events, including death.

The case for CPAP is stronger for OSA in stroke patients, and the interaction with OSA and stroke is more complicated too. OSA clearly predisposes to stroke (it more than doubles the risk) but ironically stroke seems to cause OSA in many patients who never had it before; it may appear during the immediate days and weeks following an acute stroke, and may resolve in many cases thereafter.

It is not clear why this happens, but research shows that CPAP in patients with OSA lowers stroke risk, and CPAP immediately after a stroke improves risk of future stroke and decreases the residual neurologic deficit from the stroke (physical problems, speech problems, etc.) in these patients. Once again, the problem may be worsened if the patient is not sleepy from OSA or does not feel better with CPAP, so they may be resistant to its use.

Atrial fibrillation is a rapid, irregular heart rhythm, and is another important complication of OSA. Atrial fibrillation is four times more likely in patients with untreated OSA than in normals, and the treatment and resolution of atrial fibrillation are both better with CPAP. Most atrial fibrillation patients with OSA are not sleepy, though, so the same problems with compliance may emerge.

Let's summarize what we know about CPAP:

It's very effective in eliminating OSA while it's being worn and can be adjusted to the point where OSA is completely eliminated in many cases. It can produce "miraculous" feelings in patients whose persistent sleepiness is reversed. It is cumbersome to use but many people are not bothered by this; others find this a deal-breaker.

It can improve health and prolong life in all patients, especially those with strokes and heart disease, and complete use (all-night, at best six to seven hours) appears to be much better than partial use. Lastly, success with CPAP is much more likely when a team of physicians and therapists are helping the patient in a coordinated, supportive fashion than when the patient is left to cope alone.

There are now alternatives to CPAP for treatment of OSA, some more helpful than others. *Positional sleep apnea* is diagnosed when significant obstructive events are seen only in the supine position (on one's back), and is usually only in the mildest cases. Treatment for this can be simple, using devices to prevent supine sleep. There are a number of straps, pillows, and wedges available commercially, but we found that a tennis ball affixed to the back of a T-shirt with a rubber band works fine. It's not easy to sleep on your back when you have a tennis ball pressing into your lower spine.

For mild to moderate OSA, an oral appliance (a mandibular [jaw] advancement device, or MAD) for sleep apnea can be very effective. MADs work by pushing the lower jaw forward, which pulls the back of the tongue forward and away from the back wall of the throat, preventing obstruction during sleep. Obviously, this should work better for those sleep apnea patients whose obstruction is more tongue-based than soft-palate-based.

The mandibular advancement device (MAD) is best made by a dentist specializing in sleep disorders (a sleep dentist!), after a full exam of the jaw and upper airway. The MAD is slowly adjusted over a period of days to weeks until snoring and OSA are eliminated; best practices are to use a MAD that is adjustable at home and to confirm normalization of OSA with a sleep study, usually at home, with the MAD in place.

In the 1990s and early 2000s, MADs were considered second-line therapy, to be used only if CPAP failed, but the devices and their use have improved so much that they are now first-line therapy, and many patients are offered a choice between MAD and CPAP as soon as the results of their sleep study are known.

A cheap-and-easy type of MAD is found on the internet and falls in the category of a "boil-and-bite" device. This means one buys a synthetic block which is softened in hot water and then molded to one's tooth outlines when bitten and can have some forward pressure on the jaw like the professional versions. However, these are much less effective than the prescribed, custom versions, and are really only useful for those who have snoring alone.

Now let's talk about drugs for OSA.[56] Years ago, drugs known as respiratory stimulants were tried for treatment of OSA but they seemed not to help. These drugs were known to stimulate the *drive to breathe,* which means stimulating the brain to tell the muscles of respiration to *try harder.* Wouldn't increasing that drive lessen sleep apnea? Well…not so much. These drugs did not seem to decrease the number of obstructions per hour, though they may have increased the efforts to do so. Making stronger efforts to breathe did not change the fact that the throat was obstructed during sleep. These drugs never gained much usage.

Now there is a new group of drug combinations that address nerve receptors in the soft palate* which seem to make it more sensitive to efforts to keep the airway open. None of these drugs so far results in complete reversal of sleep apnea, and none are on the market yet.

But this is a hopeful sign of things to come.

More immediately helpful and available are the GLP-1 (glucagon-like-peptide) drugs (currently with brand names like Ozempic or Mounjaro), which burst on the scene in the last few years for treatment of diabetes. Their effects on lowering blood sugar are well known, and now their ability to produce significant weight loss has been proven. Recently they have been given to OSA patients with significant improvement, all of which so far appears related to weight loss, not to any other direct effect on the airway.

We have known for years that significant weight loss in obese OSA patients (but not in skinny OSA patients like me!) can reduce or even *eliminate* OSA in many patients; the most dramatic results like this we have seen countless times in patients undergoing bariatric surgery (intestinal bypass, gastric banding, and gastric sleeve procedures, for example).

If and when the barriers—cost and insurance coverage issues, transitions from intravenous infusion to oral administration—to more universal use of GLP-1 drugs come down, it is conceivable that more than half of all OSA patients would be eligible for this approach as *first-line*

---

* Adrenergic receptors (in the sympathetic nervous system) and muscarinic receptors (in the cholinergic nervous system).

therapy, meaning something to try for OSA before CPAP, oral appliances, or HNS (hypoglossal nerve stimulation, to be discussed soon). This would be revolutionary—and has already begun.

Surgery for OSA

What about surgery? Surgery has long been available for sleep apnea, and, as we have seen, was the first available treatment for sleep apnea in the form of tracheostomy—only used as a last resort, as we have seen above, and almost never used now.

Uvulopalatopharyngoplasty

Another surgery that was done on thousands of patients in the 1990s and early 2000s was *uvulopalatopharyngoplasty*, a mouthful (sorry!) of a word, more commonly abbreviated as UPPP, or UP3. Breaking down the word, it means plastic surgery (restructuring) of the uvula, soft palate, and pharyngeal (tonsillar) walls to widen the airway in the back of the throat. There are still thousands of people in this country and worldwide who are survivors of this surgery, some with good results.

In essence, having a UP3 means having one's uvula removed and soft palate trimmed down, and sometimes the side walls of the pharynx widened with removal of tonsils. A lot of tissue is thus removed, and for those whose main site of obstruction from sleep apnea is at the soft palate level (probably 40–50% of all patients, particularly those with obesity-related sleep apnea), it could be very helpful, with significant improvement in symptoms of OSA and in the AHI, (the aforementioned apnea-hypopnea index) the main score of OSA severity. One could hope that one's OSA was "cured."

But there are problems: the postoperative pain from UP3 is said to be severe ("the worst sore throat you'll ever have"), and this led some to theorize that the postop improvement in OSA was due more to weight loss from not being able to swallow easily over the weeks after surgery than from the effects of the surgery itself. For many the improvements in sleep quality after UP3 are long-lasting, but unfortunately this is not always the case.

Indeed, for those whose OSA does improve after surgery, the good results may not last. Over the months and years postop, some patients' signs and symptoms of sleep apnea may return, and they require re-evaluation. More concerning is that in some patients the altered anatomy of the throat would allow obstruction and apnea during sleep but not snoring, so what we call "silent" apnea might occur, somewhat harder for the bedpartner to detect.

While essentially all patients who are being evaluated for UP3 have a sleep study beforehand, not all have one after, either in the immediate postop periods (say, six to 12 weeks after surgery) or long-term (say, one to two years postop.) So when further down the road we discover the return of witnessed apneas and daytime sleepiness and a repeat study shows the "return" of significant OSA, the sleep physician can't be sure if this represents a true recurrence of OSA or just a poor response to the surgery from the onset.

The lesson here is that *all patients should have a repeat sleep study after healing*, say six months postop. My thought for these patients is: Don't you want to know if you are cured?

Hypoglossal nerve stimulation

A newer procedure now available involves the hypoglossal nerve, which comes up from the base of the neck on each side and has branches that give nerve impulses to the front and back of the tongue, causing contraction of the tongue muscles. This results in forward movement of the tongue. The procedure, called hypoglossal nerve stimulation (HNS), is available today as a commercial product called "Inspire." For those who have sleep apnea with obstruction coming from the tongue base, as opposed to the soft palate, prompting the tongue to move forward during sleep to open the back of the throat may relieve that obstruction and successfully treat apnea.

HNS works well for some patients: their apneic episodes can be "dialed down" by increasing the current applied to the tongue at night, and in some cases they achieve normal results, and, more importantly, sleep better, feel better, and presumably live healthier and longer lives.[57] But since this procedure is aimed at relieving tongue-based obstruction, it's important to use it only for those patients who qualify with that kind of obstruction. The criteria for eligibility for HNS are a body mass index (BMI) of 32 or less (as heavier patients have more soft-palate obstruction, which is not relieved by HNS) and "sleep endoscopy" that visualizes a pattern of narrowing of the airway consistent with tongue-based blockage.

Of course, there are downsides to HNS, as with every procedure. It requires an operation in a surgical suite with general anesthesia for implantation, and it involves physical implantation of a signaling device, like a pacemaker, under the skin of the chest with electrodes tunneled under the skin of the neck into the tongue base on one side. Potential removal of the device requires another operation. And the basic procedure costs about *10×* more than the fitting and delivery of an oral appliance (MAD),* an apt comparison because MADs are also a good option for the same patient group: the thinner ones with tongue-based obstruction.

I have not been able to find any study of head-to-head comparison of the efficacy and outcomes of HNS compared to MAD. Both of these are convenient to use (compared to CPAP) and both have the potential for good results, but does HNS have good enough results to offset the significantly higher costs? I always advised my OSA patients to look into oral appliances first, since they are cheaper and easier to change out if there's a problem.

Other surgeries for OSA

There are a number of other surgical procedures that have been proposed for CPAP-intolerant obstructive sleep apnea. I will list their names here but will not burden you with all the anatomical and procedural details;

---

* The out-of-pocket costs to a particular patient for either approach obviously depends on the overall charges from the sleep dentist or surgeon, from the anesthesiologist and hospital, as well as the coverage for those charges by the patient's insurance company. Your mileage may vary.

some of these are still being performed, some no longer. They are *max-illomandibular advancement* (MMA), *hyoid suspension, genioglossal advancement, soft palate or tongue-base radiofrequency ablation, laser-assisted uvulopalatoplasty* (LAUP), *nasopharyngeal stents*, and others.

As CPAP and oral appliances have become more effective and easier to tolerate, the number of patients needing these second-line surgical procedures has fallen. This means that fewer such surgeries are done, which means that the average surgeon does not do many of these procedures.

Do you want to have a procedure done by someone who hasn't done many of these? I would not. So my recommendation here is that, if you need to consider surgery for sleep apnea, you may wish to seek out an experienced surgeon, someone who has done a lot of them, preferably in an academic setting.

There is another problem, though, with the surgical approach. There are many articles in the surgical literature that attest to the efficacy of each procedure—but what are the criteria for judging success?

Usually a given literature report would claim success from the procedure in any patients achieving an AHI post-op below 50% of baseline pre-op value, *or* under 20 events per hour. But this would mean, for example, that if I have sleep apnea with an AHI of 100 events per hour (very severe OSA—remember that "severe" is more than 30 per hour), and then I opt for surgery, my procedure could be deemed successful if my postop AHI is, say, 45 per hour, which is *still severe sleep apnea.*

But how is that successful? How can one claim success if the post-op results still show severe disease? The same results achieved with a CPAP or MAD would be considered a failure, and more therapy would have to be considered. In general, this led me over the years to take claims of success for surgical procedures reported in the medical literature with a good pinch of salt.

It is understandable that a person with significant OSA who cannot tolerate CPAP and/or MAD would consider surgical options. But it's important to be sure that a particular procedure is effective, and this can be done only with documentation. Again, I feel that *every patient who undergoes UP3 or any surgical procedure for OSA should have a sleep study at some appropriate interval post-op to document improvement*, and of course a sleep study later on if symptoms recur. Some surgical protocols mandate this.

I would also apply traditional criteria to success in treatment, which means achieving an overall AHI postop of (at worst) less than 15 events per hour, as this is "mild" sleep apnea and for many patients has no long-term consequences. "Optimal" would be an AHI of less than five, which is normal.

The dangers of surgery

One more thing. No discussion of obstructive sleep apnea and surgery would be complete without an explicit description of particularly high risks that *any* surgery with general anesthesia entails for many patients with OSA.

We became aware in the 1990s that something unexpected, dangerous, and sometimes tragic was happening in some people with sleep apnea when they were put to sleep for surgery. They did well in the operating room, but afterwards in the recovery room, they would not regain their own ability to breathe as expected. As a result, they would require assistance with breathing and sometimes this meant being on a ventilator for hours or even days after surgery. In some cases even cardiac arrest occurred in the recovery room, which led to transfer to the intensive care unit on a ventilator, and sometimes even death.

This is what we think happens. It appears that the breathing problems in sleep that OSA patients experience are made worse by general anesthesia, which is not a problem as long as the anesthesiologist is breathing for them in the operating room. But afterwards in the recovery room, they could not breathe on their own as OSA was closing their throats— and breathing would stop. This was, not infrequently, disastrous.

Ron was a 55-year-old bus driver who had been diagnosed with obstructive sleep apnea some years previously. His sleep study then showed an AHI (number of breathing stoppages per hour) of 66 events per hour (severe is greater than 30 per hour). He was started on CPAP early on and did very well with it, sleeping all night every night with his machine, consistently feeling more alert and awake all day. He was obese (weight 290 pounds, height 5'11", body mass index 40.4; that's severe obesity) and had hypertension and diabetes.

In 2002 he developed an inguinal hernia in the right groin, and same-day (outpatient) surgery was recommended. Although seemingly complete histories were taken by both the surgeon and the anesthesiologist before the surgery, neither asked about or were told about Ron's OSA or about his use of CPAP.

The hernia repair surgery went well. Ron was transferred to the Recovery Room post-op and, once he appeared to have regained spontaneous breathing, he was extubated [his breathing tube was removed]. Twenty minutes later, however, his oxygen levels began to fall and he appeared to be not breathing. He required re-intubation to restore breathing and was transferred to the ICU for mechanical ventilation.

Over the next few days, attempts to remove the ventilator were unsuccessful. He was finally able to breathe on his own but still required another two days in the ICU and five days in the hospital after that. At his family's insistence, his CPAP machine was used whenever he was sleeping in the ICU or in his hospital room, with good results.

The good news is that we have learned how to prevent this chain of events.[58] Preoperative screening to find any diagnosed or undiagnosed OSA is critical. In some situations regional anesthesia can be used instead of general, and the patient can have surgery but avoid being put to sleep completely. If sleep apnea is undiagnosed but suspected, evaluation by a sleep specialist before surgery can be lifesaving. With known

OSA, increased awareness immediately post-op is important, and CPAP usage immediately after surgery may prevent new respiratory failure and possibly death.

Patients with more severe OSA appear more at risk from general anesthesia, but others with less severe OSA are still vulnerable. Precautions should also be considered for anyone with OSA who is being treated with opiates or opioids, especially intravenously (as in pain therapies), as these drugs also inhibit breathing and are therefore risky for those with significant OSA.

Here are the rules I would lay down for my OSA patients before they had any general anesthesia:

- Well in advance of surgery, alert your surgeon and especially your anesthesiologist that you have OSA

- Be sure you bring your CPAP machine* with you to the hospital, and ask the anesthesiologist to commit to having it available for you in the immediate post-op time in the recovery room (not just waiting for you in your hospital room!), and from then on in the hospital until discharge

- Be sure to use CPAP *whenever you are sleeping* in the hospital (you may be receiving potent medications for pain and not know it).

Continue to use CPAP at home whenever you're sleeping.

PEARLS OF WISDOM

A diagnosis of obstructive sleep apnea is not helpful if appropriate treatment does not follow. CPAP works wonderfully for many but a team approach, with a sleep physician and sleep technicians, is more likely to result in a happy and successful outcome than anything less. Oral appliances are now first-line therapy for mild or moderate

---

* Those who use an oral appliance for OSA should follow the same rules about usage, but usually their risk of problems after surgery is lower, as this group tends to have milder OSA and fewer complications from anesthesia

sleep apnea. A board-certified sleep dentist is usually the best choice for fitting an oral appliance.

Hypoglossal nerve stimulation can also be considered as an alternative to CPAP or an oral appliance, but is more expensive and has the potential complications of surgery with general anesthesia. Other surgical options are available but considered a choice of last resort. No treatment helps if the patient is non-compliant, and a goal of at least seven hours a night with the chosen treatment is recommended. Caution is warranted whenever surgery is considered for patients with OSA.

Central sleep apnea

A number of disorders in pulmonary medicine involve "central apneas," which mean episodes of not breathing that seem to be caused by problems in the central nervous system (CNS)—as opposed to being caused by obstruction in the back of the throat, which is the case with obstructive sleep apnea. A person who suffers a high cervical spine (neck) trauma and is paralyzed from the neck down may be permanently apneic—unable to breathe, as no nerve impulses go to the intercostal muscles (between the ribs) or the diaphragm muscle, at all. These patients require mechanically assisted breathing from the beginning, just to survive.

Central sleep apnea (CSA) is a subset of these central apneas, in that the breathing problem occurs mostly or only during sleep. The most common cause of CSA is congestive heart failure (CHF), and the cause is a bit complicated.

One of the main roles of the heart is to pump blood to the lungs to pick up oxygen for delivery to the tissues for fuel, and to pick up carbon dioxide (CO_2) from the tissues as exhaust gas from energy use, and to deliver that to the lungs so it can be breathed out. When the heart begins to fail as a pump, the amount of blood pushed out with each beat begins to fall, and the amount of oxygen delivered in each beat, and the amount of CO_2 extracted from tissues both fall. Since the brain depends on blood oxygen levels and especially blood CO_2 levels as signals for how much, or how little, to ask the chest muscles to produce breathing efforts, in congestive heart failure, this system becomes unstable.

A characteristic sign of central apnea is called *periodic breathing*, where over-breathing and under-breathing are seen in a repeating pattern; this is the brain struggling to find the right level of breathing when it gets different signals from the blood. (It is like a thermostat on your wall switching on and off rapidly in trying to get the temperature in the room right.)

Periodic breathing related to CHF is more common during sleep, as CHF is frequently worse during sleep, in part because of the lying-down position. Patients with periodic breathing experience gasping and shortness of breath during sleep, causing anxiety as well as disrupted sleep. And the swings in pressures in the chest and oxygen levels in the blood can worsen heart failure, so CSA can be a vicious circle.

Remarkably, CPAP, by applying pressure to the airway with each breath, can stabilize breathing in this setting, preventing periodic breathing and thereby improving sleep quality and heart function. A variant of CPAP is called *adaptive servo-ventilation* (ASV), which uses a feedback detection of breathing to "fill in" the breaths that are missing in the under-breathing part of periodic breathing. This then stabilizes the breathing and prevents the over-breathing part too. All of this is beneficial for the heart as well.

Central apnea can be sneaky, too. It is seen in some patients with atrial fibrillation without obvious heart failure, and even some patients who are thought to have straightforward obstructive sleep apnea have evidence of central apnea on their sleep studies too.

In all these cases, CPAP or ASV may be very helpful. Close cooperation between the cardiologist and the sleep physician is critical in controlling this problem.

Central sleep apnea can cause disrupted sleep from shortness of breath and is most commonly seen in patients with heart failure and atrial fibrillation. It also occasionally complicates otherwise simple obstructive sleep apnea. Control with positive pressure breathing, like CPAP or ASV, can dramatically improve sleep and heart function.

Narcolepsy

If sleep apnea is the disease that made a specialty out of sleep medicine, it was narcolepsy that was the spark for that. Narcolepsy is the classic "sleepiness disorder"—everyone with narcolepsy is sleepy to some degree—and it was recognized as such in the 1880s in Europe. But it was not understood at all. In fact, even into the 1950s, it was considered a form of epilepsy, for reasons we will explore.

Bill Dement, the pioneering sleep researcher at Stanford, saw his first narcolepsy patient in 1958[59] and wanted to examine more, but *could not find any other doctor in the Bay Area who had seen (or at least recognized) even one such patient.* He resorted to a want-ad in the *San Francisco Chronicle* seeking people with disabling sleepiness, and quickly received 100 responses, 50 of which were from people who proved to have overt narcolepsy! He had quickly demonstrated that the disease was not rare but was vastly misunderstood and underdiagnosed.

By 1964 he had diagnosed 100 people with narcolepsy, and decided to start the world's first sleep clinic at Stanford hoping to provide care for all of them. Apparently the world was not ready for this: the clinic soon failed financially. But he continued to accrue patients, tried again, and finally made a true sleep disorders clinic viable in 1970, the world's first, aimed at diagnosing and treating all sleep disorders.

Now, as a result of his tenacity and perspicacity, there are thousands of sleep laboratories around the world.

There's an old saying in medicine that says, "When you hear hoofbeats, think of horses, not zebras." It is a way of reminding doctors at all levels of training that common things are more common than uncommon ones (duh) and the most likely diagnosis for the patient sitting in front of you is the most common illness suggested by the symptoms they have. A cold rather than leukemia, for example. (The corollary to that, of course, is never to forget all the uncommon possibilities, like leukemia too.)

When faced with a patient with daytime sleepiness, one is reminded that the most common cause of this is not narcolepsy or even sleep apnea, but *insufficient sleep*—but most patients already know if that's their problem, and don't see a doctor for that. (Occasionally I have seen a patient who was not aware that his habit of getting 51/2 hours of sleep nightly might contribute to his drowsiness and brain fogginess all day. "Real men don't need sleep!" is still a real belief among many.)

The next most common cause of abnormal daytime sleepiness is sleep apnea, as we have discussed; snoring and frequent obstructions at night can indeed be subtle and not always apparent to the patient or their bed-partner (or even their physician). One hundred times more rare than sleep apnea is narcolepsy, which places it in the realm of infrequent, but not rare or even unusual these days. (I had more than 60 narcolepsy patients in my sleep medicine practice after 30 years, and I was only one of four sleep medicine physicians at my hospital.) The number of new patients diagnosed with narcolepsy has greatly increased in proportion to all those new sleep labs in the world… all thanks to Bill Dement and his persistence in trying to start a sleep lab.

Nonetheless, even today the diagnosis of narcolepsy is typically delayed after symptoms first start, on average by about *10 years*. This is in part due to patients not always understanding that a problem exists, as well as to missed diagnoses on the part of the medical establishment.

Missy had a vague memory of not being sleepy all day before middle school, but now that she was in her 20s, it seemed she'd been sleepy her whole life. She remembered falling asleep in classes in middle and high school, and on occasion being reported by her teachers for this. Her mother had taken her to her pediatrician who suggested she get more sleep… but she felt she was already sleeping nine hours a night and still napping off and on during the day. Her high school grades suffered from her lack of alertness, and she even fell asleep during her SAT exam.

This poor performance resulted in her being denied admission to her "target" colleges; she had to settle for one of her "safeties." In college she struggled to stay awake in classes and did not perform to her own grade standards; she knew she could do better. Coffee helped her sleepiness—a little. A friend with ADHD gave her one of her Adderall tablets, and this helped a lot, but the effect did not last and her friend could not share any more medicines.

Missy's roommate during her sophomore year, Beth, had a sparkling personality and a great sense of humor. She loved jokes, as did Missy. But Missy began to notice a profound sense of weakness in her neck and shoulders when she laughed hard at one of Beth's jokes; sometimes her knees felt weak too, and on one occasion she actually fell to the floor while laughing. Beth took this as a compliment to the hilarity of her stories, but Missy worried that it meant something else. The weakness usually resolved in a few minutes.

In her senior year she began having nightmares, sometimes with a very real sense that someone was in her dorm room who meant to do her harm; once she was convinced that she saw someone at the foot of the bed, someone who… wasn't there. On other occasions she woke early in the morning with the sense that she could not move or speak, though she knew she was awake. These episodes were rare but disturbing.

In her senior year Missy fell asleep while driving home for Christmas vacation, a single-car accident that resulted in a brief hospitalization for a concussion. This got everyone's attention, and triggered a series of medical examinations at home, but nothing other than daytime sleepiness was found. A sleep specialist was consulted.

The sleep specialist suspected narcolepsy, and ordered an overnight sleep study, to be followed by a multiple sleep latency test (MSLT). The overnight sleep study showed a short sleep latency (she

*fell asleep within four minutes of lights out—normal is over 15 min-
utes), and REM sleep was recorded very early in the session (which
is suggestive of narcolepsy). No sleep apnea was seen.*

*The MSLT, a series of short naps in the sleep lab during the fol-
lowing day, showed an average sleep latency (time to fall asleep)
of 2.5 minutes over five naps, and REM was seen early in three of
these naps. Based on her history and the sleep studies, a diagnosis
of type 1 narcolepsy with cataplexy, sleep paralysis, and hypnogogic
hallucinations (see below) was made.*

*She improved dramatically with medical treatment, and sub-
sequently graduated magna cum laude in biology from graduate
school. She is now considering medical school.*

Narcolepsy is now understood to be a disorder of the nerve cells in
the hypothalamus that produce a peptide* called *hypocretin* or *orexin*.
(The peptide was discovered in 1998 by researchers on both sides of the
country almost simultaneously, and the two names they were given are
still used interchangeably.) Our current understanding of the functions
of orexin (I'll stick with this name) are many, but importantly includes
promoting wakefulness and the stabilization of sleep stages, so that defi-
ciencies of orexin may result in "flipping" between stages, as between
wake and sleep, and intermixing of stages, as in mixtures of wake and
REM—as well as daytime sleepiness, often profound.

Low levels of orexin in the CSF (cerebrospinal fluid) correlate with
severe narcolepsy, but taking CSF for analysis, as in a spinal tap, is a
somewhat risky and uncomfortable procedure, so it is rarely done clini-
cally. Low orexin levels also occur when the patient has *cataplexy*, a fascinating symptom which has confused physicians in previous decades,
leading to misdiagnosis.

Cataplexy is the sudden onset of muscle weakness, either localized
(usually from the neck up) or generalized, in the presence of certain

---

* A peptide is a short chain of amino acids that make up the building blocks of
proteins.

emotions such as laughter, anger, or surprise. A patient with narcolepsy and cataplexy when told a joke may notice difficulty holding up their head, keeping their mouth closed, having their shoulders slump, or in generalized cases having their knees buckle and then falling to the ground. These spells last only one to three minutes and then resolve completely. The patient is awake throughout.

The weakness can be intermittent, in an on-off-on-off pattern, so an observer might see twitches as the muscles regain and then lose again their tone multiple times during the event. It is these twitches that have caused decades of misdiagnosis of narcolepsy as seizures. This is *not epilepsy* and is not related to seizures. Cataplexy appears to be from wake/REM mixing—the sleep stage "destabilization" we mentioned above.

In cataplexy, aspects of REM sleep may suddenly occur during wakefulness, and part of that REM sleep is the weakness arising from the normal paralysis we all experience in REM. Why does this happen in emotional situations? This is not yet well understood, but there are clues that it may involve dopamine levels in the amygdala—which makes sense: the amygdala is one of the "arbiters of emotions" in the brain, and dopamine is related to reward and pleasure, which can arise, for example, with laughter.

Cataplexy is the key to diagnosing type 1 narcolepsy (called NT1). NT1 is considered more severe than type 2 (NT2), where there is no cataplexy, and where the CSF orexin level is usually normal. Whenever a person is suspected of having narcolepsy, a diligent search for cataplexy usually occurs, looking for obvious or sometimes very subtle examples of episodic weakness. If cataplexy is confidently found, a diagnosis of NT1 is assured; otherwise NT2 is likely. Occasionally cataplexy starts some months or years after NT2 is diagnosed, and the patient is then re-categorized as NT1.

Narcoleptics always experience sleepiness, sometimes with *sleep attacks*, related apparently to sleep disruption at night and slipping *suddenly* into sleep (sometimes right into REM) from wakefulness during the day. Overall the 24-hour amount of sleep is still normal. Sleepiness and sleep attacks can be dangerous and disabling, and cause accidents, school and job problems, and mood disorders.

The other important symptoms are *hallucinations* and *sleep paralysis.* (Not every narcoleptic gets all these symptoms.) Hallucinations can occur at the beginning or at the end of sleep and appear to be a wake/REM mixture, so wakeful dreaming—an hallucinatory experience—is occurring. The hallucinations may be visual but can also be auditory (hearing voices or sounds) or tactile (feeling sensations, like touch) and may confuse a physician into thinking the patient is in a psychotic episode.

Sleep paralysis occurs when the patient wakes from sleep, is convinced that they are awake, but is aware that they cannot move a muscle. Both the hallucinations of narcolepsy and sleep paralysis are more manifestations of sleep stage destabilization—wake/REM mixing—as in cataplexy above. In both cases, a characteristic of REM (dreaming in the case of hallucinations, normal muscle paralysis in the case of sleep paralysis) are mixing with the consciousness of wake. Both of these states can be disturbing for the patient, especially if they do not understand why they are happening.

One fascinating aspect of sleep paralysis is that the episode ends if the person is touched or spoken to by another, which is thought to be the origin of the *Sleeping Beauty* fairy tale: she was awakened from her unending slumber by a kiss. True sleep paralysis lasts only a few minutes; it also occurs in 7% of normals (I have had it a few times).

The onset of narcolepsy is typically in adolescence, most commonly around age 11–15; there is another peak in incidence around age 30. Occasionally much younger and much older people are diagnosed. Recently a strong association with *influenza A* has been found, with a dramatic increase in childhood cases a few months after the H1N1 flu pandemic in 2009. Some patients also have high antibody levels to the *streptococcus* bacterium, as *strep* infections may typically follow the flu.

These and other immune data suggest that narcolepsy may be an autoimmune disease, with the immune system confusing orexin-producing nerve cells with viral antigens, and attacking both. Attempts at standard treatments for immune diseases, as with steroids or infused immuno-globulins, so far have not been helpful. Given the dramatic progress made against other autoimmune diseases, such as inflammatory bowel disease, using "biologics" that alter specific parts of the immune system, there is hope for better narcolepsy treatments in the future.

Narcolepsy is diagnosed with an overnight sleep study, followed by an MSLT (see page 59). The overnight study serves to confirm adequate sleep the night before the MSLT, and to look for any other cause of sleepiness, such as sleep apnea. The MSLT is a multiple-nap study which is always done after an overnight study–it is never done by itself. The MSLT looks for rapid sleep onset (short sleep latency) in each nap and for REM onsets during those naps. Normal sleepers don't show any episodes of REM (called "REM onsets") at all in a 20-minute nap opportunity.

If the patient has nothing abnormal on the test the night before and has a short sleep latency (an average during the naps of less than eight minutes) and two or more REM onsets, they are diagnosed with NT1 (if they also have cataplexy) or NT2 (if they don't). Short sleep latency on MSLT is called "pathologic sleepiness" by testing criteria; if this is present but no REM onsets are present, the diagnosis of *idiopathic hypersomnia* is considered—more on that below.

These diagnostic criteria can be confusing. Let's look at some examples:

Michael, a 26-year-old graduate student, is being evaluated for daytime sleepiness he has experienced since middle school. Here are some variations on his testing results and the consequent diagnoses:

1. *His history and sleep diaries (sleep times recorded by him at home) suggest that he is averaging five hours of sleep nightly. A trial of increasing his overnight sleep times dramatically improves his daytime sleepiness. A diagnosis of insufficient sleep is made, and no laboratory testing is done.*

2. *His sleep diaries suggest that he is getting sufficient overnight sleep. An overnight sleep study is normal. An MSLT the following day shows an average fall-asleep time (sleep latency) of 3.5 minutes over five naps (normal is more than eight minutes). REM*

onsets are seen in three naps. The diagnosis is narcolepsy as a cause of his pathologic sleepiness, and will be called type 1 (NT1) if he has a history of cataplexy, or type 2 (NT2) if he does not.

3. *He appears to be getting sufficient overnight sleep. His overnight sleep study is normal. An MSLT the following day shows an average sleep latency of 3.5 minutes over five naps. No REM onsets are seen. The diagnosis is not narcolepsy (must have REM onsets!), but instead idiopathic hypersomnia as the cause of his pathologic sleepiness.*

4. *He appears to be getting sufficient overnight sleep. His overnight sleep study shows mild sleep apnea. An MSLT the following day shows an average fall-asleep time (sleep latency) of 3.5 minutes over five naps. No REM onsets are seen. The diagnosis is sleep apnea as the cause of his pathologic sleepiness.* *

Narcolepsy is a lifelong problem. For those with cataplexy, it is encouraging to hear that this seems to improve over time, though not in everyone.

Advice to those with newly-diagnosed narcolepsy, frequently those in their teens and 20s, includes good sleep hygiene (lots of attention to good sleep hours and habits) and often "prescribed naps." Sleepiness in narcolepsy often responds dramatically to short naps (no longer than 20 to 30 minutes), with a sense of being refreshed lasting sometimes for hours after. One or two short naps a day may allow some patients to avoid or minimize medication. Patients benefit when doctors certify the need for naps to schools or employers, who may appreciate the subsequent improved alertness and output from their student or employee.

---

* Occasionally a person has both sleep apnea and narcolepsy. The narcolepsy part can be diagnosed once the treatment of OSA is in place (for example, the patient is sleeping with CPAP) during a subsequent overnight sleep study and MSLT. If the results as in (2) above are found, then a diagnosis of both sleep apnea and narcolepsy is made.

Good sleep habits are also critical in improving daytime alertness. Regular sleep hours and minimal use of alcohol and avoidance of recreational drugs are keys to controlling narcolepsy.

The medical treatment of narcolepsy has been aimed at improving sleepiness and cataplexy. The most commonly used medications are *stimulant drugs*, such as amphetamines (such as Adderall), Ritalin, and more recently *alerting drugs*, such as modafinil (Provigil) and armodafinil (Nuvigil). These last two are intended to produce alertness while avoiding the nervousness and rapid pulse that stimulants can cause, and importantly without the potential for abuse. These drugs have helped thousands of patients with NT1 and NT2.

Another approach involves *histamine*. It is not surprising to hear that histamine is an alerting neurotransmitter in the brain, once one remembers how powerfully *antihistamines* (like Benadryl) produce sleepiness, and in fact comprise the bestselling group of over-the-counter sleeping medications in the world. Some of the newer drugs for narcolepsy operate on the concept that histamine-like medications will improve alertness, and for many patients these are helpful.

Sodium oxybate (Xyrem) is in a class of its own. We have all heard of the "date-rape" drug, sometimes slipped into the drinks of unsuspecting females. This is GHB (gamma hydroxybutyric acid), in its villainous role; it produces sleepiness and even unconsciousness, leaving one vulnerable to another's inappropriate behavior. Sodium oxybate is a chemical variant of GHB, and, given its criminal history, its use and dosing are now strictly regulated by the FDA, utilizing special pharmacies.

Why would a medication that drugs a person into unconsciousness be useful for those who are already too sleepy? It's not completely clear, but it may have to do with the disrupted sleep that is characteristic of narcolepsy, which in itself may contribute to daytime sleepiness. Sodium oxybate may deepen sleep—it actually increases delta (N3) sleep—and seems to improve this sleep disruption, decreasing awakenings and thereby improving daytime sleepiness. Effects on REM are variable.

It also decreases cataplexy, a big benefit. This may be a daytime effect of a nighttime drug, possibly occurring by decreasing the wake/REM mixing that constitutes cataplexy, as we discussed above.

Care must be taken with sodium oxybate in patients who have social reasons to need to be awakened at night, such as those who have to respond to small children, or those on night call, like doctors or EMTs. For some people this medication is a godsend; for others, a nonstarter.

Theoretically, the most appropriate medication treatment for narcolepsy, an orexin deficiency, would be replacement of orexin, but that has proved to be difficult. Orexin has been given orally, intravenously, intranasally, and even directly into the brain (in animal models of narcolepsy) with poor results. This is because orexin is not transported well across the blood-brain barrier and, within the brain, is broken down rapidly. There is hope, however, as newer drugs that attach to orexin receptors ("orexin agonists") are showing promise and are in human trials.

If this class of drugs helps those with true orexin deficiency (NT1), what about those with narcolepsy but no orexin deficiency (NT2)? It seems that either NT2 patients will improve with this replacement therapy, in which case more questions will arise about what true "orexin deficiency" means (could one have normal levels but a more non-functioning orexin?). Or, if there is no improvement, more questions will be asked about the real relationship between NT1 and NT2: are they really the same disease in different levels of severity, or just different? Either way, in the long run, progress will continue.

PEARLS OF WISDOM

Narcolepsy is an important cause of daytime sleepiness. It is sad that the diagnosis is usually delayed by many years after symptoms start, as the disorder should be considered early, especially in teens who are persistently sleepy. Good sleep habits and treatment with alerting medications can be life-changing.

Idiopathic hypersomnia

"Idiopathic hypersomnia" means "sleepiness we don't understand," and remarkably this has become the formal name for this disorder.

Idiopathic hypersomnia is the red-headed stepchild of the central hypersomnias. Central hypersomnias are the sleepiness disorders that arise from the CNS (the central nervous system), which clearly includes NT1 and NT2 above, given what we know about orexin and sleep stage irregularities of the CNS in those patients.

I know of no other disease name in modern parlance that is this vague. There are, for example, no diseases in dermatology formally called "confusing rash," or in cardiology any disorder called "perplexing heart problem." In the past, names to replace "idiopathic hypersomnia" such as "functional hypersomnia" and "harmonious hypersomnia" were considered, but never adopted. If research ever gives us firmer information on its pathophysiology, it might no longer be "idiopathic," and would require renaming.

Be that as it may, idiopathic hypersomnia (IHS) is diagnosed at least as commonly as narcolepsy, and is as disabling for some as is moderate narcolepsy. It comes in two flavors: sleepiness alone, or sleepiness with long sleep times (sometimes 10 to 12 hours of sleep nightly), and is associated with "sleep inertia"—which means difficulty waking up completely, struggling to shake off that feeling of sleepiness, sometimes for hours—and "sleep drunkenness"—which means *really* having trouble waking up. The two types, with or without long sleep time, are now considered the same illness. It most commonly affects those 10–30 years old, and more women than men.

IHS causes sleepiness but usually not "sleep attacks," as narcolepsy can do. It is usually not related to other facets of narcolepsy such as hallucinations or sleep paralysis, and by definition never involves cataplexy (which defines narcolepsy, specifically NT1). IHS does not appear related to weak sleep stage boundaries as is narcolepsy. The sleepiness can be disabling, though, as in narcolepsy.

The diagnosis is confirmed by the overnight sleep study followed by an MSLT. In IHS, no cause for sleepiness is found on the overnight study, and no more than one early REM onset is seen during the study or the naps of the MSLT. Pathologic sleepiness is the only significant finding, with a mean sleep latency of less than eight minutes averaged over those naps.

Patients with IHS are encouraged to maintain good sleep habits but many are already sleeping more than usual. Short naps are not prescribed as they give little benefit (this is a helpful diagnostic clue suggesting that narcolepsy is absent).

Continued observation of patients with IHS is warranted, as the diagnosis may change with time. Some patients go on to show evidence of narcolepsy instead (usually the mild version, NT2) and a small percentage (17% in one study) may have complete resolution of symptoms: it just goes away.[60] How nice for them!

The medications used to reverse the sleepiness of IHS are the same stimulant and alerting medications used in narcolepsy, and these work well. The irony is that, except, with the exception of low-sodium oxybate (LSO), none of them are approved for use by the FDA for IHS, though they are approved for narcolepsy. This means that these drugs are frequently used "off-label" for IHS, as they should be, given that the medical literature supports their use in IHS just as in narcolepsy. Insurance coverage for these and other nonapproved drugs for IHS may be a problem, given the lack of FDA approval.

Antidepressants and remarkably, an antibiotic (clarithromycin) have been used in some success, but no one drug helps everyone. Sodium oxybate has also been used for IHS, with partial success, and the newer sodium-limited version of sodium oxybate has shown enough success to gain FDA approval in 2021; it is now the only drug approved for this disorder, which makes no sense.

One might ask if there is a relationship between IHS and "tiredness" diseases like chronic fatigue syndrome and fibromyalgia. It is sometimes difficult to differentiate between "sleepiness" and "fatigue," though we think of fatigue as a tiredness that does not seem to respond to sleep, whereas we think of sleepiness as always begging for more sleep, and usually feeling better after sleep. Also, chronic fatigue and fibromyalgia patients usually have somatic symptoms (like headache and muscle aches) and may even complain of insomnia. Nonetheless, sleep studies will be necessary to clarify the situation.

To say that IHS is the redheaded stepchild of the sleepiness diseases is not to say it does not get a lot of attention; research continues in many places, and optimism for progress is justified. This is one more disease that no one knew *even existed* a few decades ago; let's hope that enough will be learned about it in the future to allow us treat those people who have it more effectively, not to mention to award it a real name.

PEARLS OF WISDOM

Idiopathic hypersomnia, like narcolepsy, is an important cause of daytime sleepiness. Anyone with persistent daytime sleepiness should be screened for this. Treatment can be life-changing. Unlike narcolepsy, idiopathic hypersomnia may, in some people, resolve over many years' time.

Circadian rhythm disorders

Circadian rhythm disorders are not uncommon. One type that affects everyone in this country is the clock-time change we perform almost everywhere in this country twice a year ("spring forward, fall back," as the saying goes). We may not feel much effect from that one hour of time change, though there are dat[61] suggesting more risks than one might think. But the circadian rhythm problem most people associate with symptoms is *jet lag*, a problem that did not exist before the Wright brothers made their mark on civilization.

Jet lag

If you've ever experienced jet lag—if you've ever crossed a number of time zones in a short time and then had problems with sleepiness and/or insomnia as a result, you have had a circadian rhythm disorder. Circadian rhythm (CR) problems are all variants of jet lag; the main difference is that jet lag goes away in a few days, if you stop changing time zones, while other classic circadian rhythm disorders persist until they are treated.

If you fly from New York in the Eastern Standard Time zone (EST) to, say, Paris, you will have crossed six time zones quickly. That's the setup for jet lag. At first your brain thinks you are still in the EST, so when it's 10am in Paris it's only 4am back home (where your brain still resides), so you will feel sleepy; when it's 10pm in Paris and you consider going to bed, your brain think it's only 4pm, so you may have trouble falling asleep.

Remember from our discussion of circadian rhythms that the time-setters—the things that daily reset one's CR—are, in order of strength: light, melatonin, and social activity. What will improve your jet lag in Paris is exposure to sunlight and, to a lesser extent, your social activities (such as dining) on Paris time. And if you take melatonin properly, your CR may reset faster.

In essence, by flying east you have induced a *delay* in your sleep phase (the timing of your sleep hours); at first your brain still wants to sleep 10pm to 6am EST, which now, in Paris, is 4am to noon (Paris time). You will have trouble sleeping in Paris until 4am but after noon you have trouble staying awake. Morning sunlight will help decrease the six-hour delay over the next few days, until your normal CR aligns with Paris time. You will feel normal for the rest of your trip.

Then you fly back to New York. You just came from Paris time so in NYC on EST when it's 4pm your brain thinks it's 10pm, and now you've induced a sleep phase *advance*. Now when 4pm EST comes around on the day of your arrival in New York, your brain feels it's 10pm, and *wham!* You're sleepy. If you surrender to the temptation to sleep, you will awaken at midnight EST (which is 6am Paris time, your brain time) and will sleep no more. Once again, eventually sunlight and activities will re-align you with your local EST.

What is the best way to prevent jet lag? This is perhaps more difficult than it might seem. Over a period of years, I tried a number of methods, none of which were entirely satisfactory. One approach is to pretreat for jet lag by adapting to the destination time before leaving. Then once one arrives, one has already converted to the new time zone. In the Paris example, this would mean going to sleep at home earlier and earlier, and getting up earlier and earlier, in the days preceding leaving for Paris.

Let's say you live in New York and are travelling to Paris in two weeks. To mimic Paris time while in New York, you would gradually advance your sleep phase from your usual 10pm-to-6am EST pattern to a target 4pm-to-2am EST; this target aims to mimic 10pm-to-4pm Paris time. By the time you board the plane to leave NYC, you are already on Paris time. If you board at 5pm EST, your brain is already "in" Paris where it is 11pm, and you can sleep until landing. And when you do land in Paris at 7am Paris time, even though it's actually 1am in NYC, your brain is already adjusted to 7am Paris time and you are ready for the day. *Voilà!* No jet lag!

But the cost of this approach is not insignificant. Going to bed earlier and earlier, until eventually one is retiring six hours before one's usual bedtime, is hard. It's harder to get to sleep earlier and earlier, and it restricts, eventually severely, one's evening activities, such as family interactions and meals. Getting to bed earlier and earlier, eventually as early as 4pm, may be impossible for someone with a job or other daily responsibilities where one might not normally be home yet by that time.

And while getting up earlier and earlier, as early as 2am, may not be as difficult, if one has truly slept for 7–8 hours as planned, what does one do in those early morning hours when everyone else is asleep? Read? Play on the computer? Work at home? This can feel strange, like time wasted, having to wait long hours before the sun comes up and one can go to work or school, and feeling *a bit off* all that time from the sleep time changes.

Plus, like many people, I usually find myself unable to sleep on the plane. This is a problem many of us have, particularly when First-Class, lying-down seats are not in one's budget, as Economy seats do not promote normal sleep, to say the least. Instead, they are a formula for insomnia. Some can overcome this with sleeping pills, but these do not work for many (including me), so a night of almost complete wakefulness on the plane can undo a week of diligent time-shifting to avoid jet lag, and one can arrive at destination feeling worse than ever. Not a great result.

My daughter, 12 years old at the time, agreed to try time zone shifting with me years ago before a trip to France. We moved our bedtimes and wake times back gradually in the week before the trip, not easy as I was working and she was in school. Then on the flight to Paris, she fell asleep—and I didn't. At all, it seemed. There was a connecting flight the next day to Toulouse, but still no sleep for me. Picking up our rental car in Toulouse, I backed into a post—clearly visible behind the car as we loaded our luggage—and put a one-inch hole in the fender of a brand-new BMW. My wife tells me this was the first time my children had ever heard me swear. I attribute that misadventure to acute sleep deprivation with the attention deficit that this causes. I was not a happy camper and dreaded returning the car at the end of the trip.*

There are other ways to shift one's time zone, using carefully timed melatonin and/or bright line administration. I have tried all of these approaches, and also tried reversing them on the trips back. But eventually I arrived at a realization: I was trying to make my trip better, by forcing my brain to adapt to my destination before I left—while my body was still at home. Going to bed earlier and earlier was disruptive to my home and work life, and I slept less well in this earlier (advanced) sleep phase. Getting up earlier and earlier meant I was going to work after many more hours of wakefulness than usual, so I began to feel sleepier at work. For over a week before the trip, I felt worse and worse.

---

* They didn't charge me much. I love the French.

I have concluded that a week of forcing myself to feel terrible, with family and job disruption, as a trade-off for perhaps two days at destination with jet lag, is not worth the effort. Now I just plan that the first day or so on the trip will be difficult but will improve with time. That is not true for everyone, though: some people say that a simple sleeping pill, like Lunesta, taken once at bedtime on the plane, makes them feel rested on arrival and mitigates jet lag.

Others have more success with some abbreviated form of adaptation to the one I have described. But given how well we understand jet lag now, and how many suggestions one can find on the internet for how to prevent it, it's telling that there is no one well-accepted way to do that, which tells me there's no really successful way to achieve that. We just have to find what works for us.

There are a number of apps online that help with advice about when to use or avoid light, darkness, caffeine, and alcohol to adapt to particular time-zone crossings. These can be very helpful in choosing behavioral changes before or after travel but can still be derailed if good sleep quality and quantity on the plane is necessary—which it usually is. In jet lag considerations, we say "East is least and west is best," meaning that it's easier to fly west during the day and then sleep when you arrive in a bed than to sleep on the plane sitting up going east and staying up when you arrive. That's because our circadian rhythms tolerate lengthening better than shortening (our normal rhythm is a bit more than 24 hours, remember?), and flying west means a longer first day, flying east a shorter one.

Either way, the rule of thumb for normal CR adaptation is 1.5 time zones a day, which means that when you fly to California from the east coast and cross three time zones, you will recover from jet lag in two days just with normal activity (light and social activity at the normal times for your destination). Crossing six time zones to get to Paris makes this a less pleasant four-day adaptation. In my experience, I'm almost normal after two days.

If you want to try to prevent jet lag on your next travel across time zones, calculate how many hours difference your destination is from your current time zone, and try shifting your sleep times gradually, over a week or so, to match that—going to bed earlier for travel east, later for travel west—and see if you can make that work. If you are able to sleep well on the plane on the way, all the better. Some people can do this quite successfully, but I am not one of those. I hope you are!

Shiftwork sleep disorder

People who work during night (dark) hours may have difficulty staying awake during that time as well as problems sleeping during the off (day) hours. "Shift work disorder" arises when work periods are outside the normal hours of wakefulness, traditionally outside the "normal" daytime hours. We know from our understanding of circadian rhythms that the brain will object to sleep–wake patterns that don't fit one's normal rhythms, that demand wake when we want sleep, and vice versa. Nontraditional shift work hours can lead to difficulty sleeping during the desired sleep time and difficulty staying awake during the working hours, which can be annoying, problematic, and even dangerous.

Evening shift work (say, working from 4pm to midnight) pushes these boundaries slightly, but may be palatable or even preferable for those with a "night owl" chronotype—those who function better if they stay up later and sleep later than normals (see page 41). Others, especially "morning larks" like me, who tend to go to bed earlier and get up earlier, struggle with evening shifts.

Obviously, night shifts (say, starting work at 11pm and clocking off at 7am) create the biggest circadian rhythm problem for most people, no matter what their circadian chronotype. "Rotating shifts" are also problematic—involving working days, then evenings, then nights, or some other sequence, changing every few days or weeks. As necessary as it may be to have health, emergency, law-enforcement, and other workers stay up to work at night, the toll these "anti-rhythms" take on those workers is difficult to avoid. It's a toss-up whether the "brain scramble" that comes from continuous night shift work is worse that the scramble/unscramble/re-scramble that come from rotating shifts.

In a perfect world, workers would be chosen for particular shifts depending on their chronotypes: night owls would be selected for evening shifts, morning larks for daytime shifts. In reality, some self-select for the work times with which they're most comfortable. But few people are drawn to or can adapt perfectly to continuous night shift work, with its demands for alertness during the dark hours and sleeping during the day.

And what to do about weekends or days off? Rotate to sleeping at night, awake during the day? That's hard to do when the next group of night shifts is coming up, say, two days later. Continue to sleep days, stay awake nights on days off? Then one misses out on social interaction with the rest of the world. It's a big dilemma.

Larry and Mo both worked night shifts at Amazon, with very demanding work processing packages between 11pm and 7am every night. A work-week was Monday night through Friday night, with Saturday and Sunday nights off. Both came to me with problems sleeping during the day after work, so we instituted a standard plan (see below) with bright light in the evenings before work and darkness and quiet at home for daytime sleep. This worked well for both.

But they differed in how they wanted to deal with their time off. Larry wanted to have normal wake hours on the weekends to spend with his girlfriend; this meant coming home from Friday night work on Saturday morning and staying up all day Saturday, sleeping Saturday night normally, and doing the same on Sunday. We used more bright light on Saturday and Sunday mornings to help him stay awake, a melatonin supplement at bedtime with good bedroom protection Saturday and Sunday nights. This worked for his weekends but Mondays were still difficult, as he would be awake all day Monday then stay awake all Monday night at work, so a nap was built into his Monday evenings before work. None of this was optimal (shiftwork therapy rarely is) but it worked better for him.

Mo was easier. He had no girlfriend and was happy to sleep on weekends during the day just as he did during the week, and he liked being up all night at home on Saturdays and Sundays. We did not have to change his routine on weekends.

Shift work disorder involves missing nighttime sleep, and, for most, getting less than optimal sleep during the day. It's a form of chronic sleep deprivation, and as such is not surprisingly associated with higher risks of inappropriate sleepiness with consequent errors of judgment, mood problems, and vehicle accidents, as well as more risk of glucose intolerance, diabetes, metabolic and cardiovascular disease, and even cancer.[62]

For those working evening shifts, it may suffice to shift sleep times later. Working 3–11pm might still allow normal sleep time from midnight to 8am, or 1am to 9am (depending on commute times), which would minimize circadian disruption, especially for night-owls, and promote daytime and work-time alertness.

Night-shift work is, of course, harder. To work, for example, from 11pm to 7am requires efforts to remain awake and alert throughout the traditional sleeping hours in the dark and to sleep during the day, in the traditional sleep hours. This goes against the grain of the patterns that our circadian rhythms have evolved for us. Try adapting to this schedule for two weeks and you'll likely have persistent problems with insomnia during the day and problems with sleepiness and attention deficits during your work hours at night.

We can apply some circadian rhythm principles to this problem, knowing what we know about light and phase shifts. We want to be awake all night? Then we stay in bright light in the hours before work in the evening, and get a burst of bright light before work begins, using a light box (see page 85); this uses light to inhibit the normal output of melatonin that occurs in the evening, helping to prevent sleepiness. A bright light environment throughout the nighttime work hours will also help (though it may be harmful to those around us, such as patients in the ICU, who need their sleep).

On our way home from work in the morning, we want to avoid bright light as much as possible, wearing dark glasses while driving from work if it's after dawn and keeping dim light at home until we can crawl into bed. We put a sign on our doorbell saying "Day Sleeper: Please do not ring," silence our phones, and use blackout curtains in our bedroom. All this is to optimize sleep chances by minimizing light exposure and welcoming melatonin output from the darkness we enjoy. We hope to shift our circadian rhythms to better synchronize with the night shift pattern.

Some have advocated sleeping pills (such as benzodiazepines, not my favorites) for the day sleeper. Since there may be persistent sleepiness that carries over into the work period at night, this may not be a good idea. Low-dose (0.5–2.0mg) melatonin makes more sense, to be taken on arrival home, which may have less of the hangover effect.

What many shiftworkers do is muddle through, trying to adjust to day-wake and night-sleep for just two days. Since circadian shifts move slowly, using bright light and melatonin to shift back in just two days does not make sense, and may worsen adaptation to going back to night shift work after the weekend.

My long-term recommendation for the night shift group is the same as what most of my patients told me they had already decided: to work through merit and seniority (and pressure, if it helps) within their companies to earn the preferred day or evening shifts. Work hard and earn your spot, and be a squeaky wheel. Your brain will thank you.

Other circadian rhythm disorders

Another common formal circadian rhythm sleep problem is *delayed sleep phase syndrome* (DSPS), which commonly affects those in their teens and 20s sometimes later. The other is *advanced sleep phase syndrome* (ASPS) which is seen mainly in older patients.

Let's discuss the common delayed version first.

It's helpful to understand that *a normal delay in sleep phase occurs in all adolescents*. All children going through puberty develop a tendency to have later bedtimes and later wake times, and this has been shown to occur mostly independent of social activity (such as staying up late on the phone, computer, or watching TV). In fact, a close correlation between sleep phase delay and formal (Tanner) stages of puberty have been shown, which means that as different aspects of normal puberty make themselves known (like degree of pubic hair growth), the amount of sleep phase delay (in minutes) increases.

All adolescents are now recognized as having the normal need to go to sleep later and wake later than their younger selves, which means it may be harder for them to be awake at their usual times at the beginning of the school day.

A child who before puberty would easily fall asleep at 9pm and wake at 6am will after, say, age 13 normally shift to a phase with sleepiness beginning at 11pm and waking at 8am. This amounts to a two-hour shift in the phase, sometimes to the great surprise of their parents. You can see that this does not work well if the child has to be at school at 7am; sleeping, or at best just sleepiness, in the first morning classes may result. For this reason a grassroots movement to make middle school starting times later has been successful in some states and countries, and has resulted in improved grades, less tardiness and absences, less depression, and in young drivers, fewer accidents.[63]

But if a delayed phase is normal in children and teens, why are we all, as adults, not still delayed? Because the process seems to resolve in the late teens or early 20s, with the sleep phase "advancing" back to a normal time slowly during those years. The occasional person in their 20s or even 30s will not revert for some reason and will complain of not being able to sleep until 2–3am in some cases, and not wanting to wake until 10am to noon. (See **Figure 4B**, page 180.)

This is a very delayed sleep phase and constitutes delayed sleep phase syndrome. It can be devastating for one's work or social life, not to mention leading to problems of sleep deprivation when the sleep needs of this phase cannot be met, when one simply can't stay in bed until mid-day because of work demands, for example. All the problems of sleep deprivation then occur.

Some DSPS patients can adjust using just *chronotherapy.* This means incrementally moving their voluntary sleep times and rising times forward (it's easier forward than backward) until they are at an acceptable phase.

Stephen, a 23-year-old landscaper, tried chronotherapy a few years ago. Like many untreated DSPS patients he found that he could not go to sleep before 3am and therefore needed to sleep until 11am every day. This was incompatible with his life and work hours. We decided that he would use an upcoming two weeks of vacation to try chronotherapy.

For his two nights, I asked him to fight sleep at his usual 3am bedtime, to resist going to bed until 5am. He was allowed to get up from bed when he felt rested. His bedtime was moved by two hours every two nights, so after 10 nights of shifting, he was set to go to bed at 11pm—which is what he wanted. He had no problem getting eight hours of sleep on all these nights, so his eventual rising time was 7am, which was great for him.

This worked great for him for months. But then he was invited to a weekend house party, and found himself staying up well after midnight for multiple nights. When he returned home he found he was back to his old pattern of bedtime 3am, risetime 11am, and his work hours again were threatened. When this did not resolve, we found another time to use chronotherapy again, and he has done well since.

Chronotherapy works well for many, resetting them from a very late bedtime to a normal one, one that works with their lifestyle. But if they are not careful, if they stay up late for a night or two, they lose their new-found pattern altogether and revert to a delayed phase again. They may have to start all over. As you can imagine, the process of time-shifting with chronotherapy is disruptive to daily life during the changeover, so we try to find downtime or vacation time from work for the patient to go through this process.

More resistant DSPS can be treated with bright light and melatonin. Both of these, given at the precise right times (morning for the light, evening for the melatonin) will advance the phase back toward normal. The details of the light and melatonin (exact amounts and timing of each) must be correct for this to work. Successful re-alignment of the circadian rhythm (CR) is almost always achieved this way.

Commercial light boxes can provide the necessary 10,000 lux (a measure of brightness) for 30 minutes at the exact right time every morning, and melatonin is given at the precise evening time calculated to move the CR by one to two hours each night.

The typical patient with delayed sleep phase syndrome (DSPS) is in their late teens or early 20s by the time they are diagnosed and treated. They do very well if they stick with the program, rejoining the main body of the human race who get sleepy at night and wake in the mornings at "normal" times. Success with this is very gratifying for both patient and physician.

Another "normal" circadian rhythm change occurs in most of the elderly: sleep phase advance, known as *advanced sleep phase syndrome* (ASPS), which is the tendency to become sleepy earlier than usual and wake earlier than usual—with the overall number of sleep hours unchanged. (See **Figure 4C,** page 180.) This is why you see so many elderly people at the Early Bird Special at your local cafeteria; dinner at 5:30pm, home by 7pm and in bed by 8pm is not unusual, with wake around 4–5am for some being a habit.

Since many of these older people are retired and freed from the demands of school and work, they may not complain of this problem. But when it is severe and disabling, interfering with social life or work, or when it occurs in younger (middle-aged) patients, it can be treated if necessary with bright light (in the evenings) and melatonin (in the mornings).

Two other recognized circadian rhythm disorders are *non-24-hour sleep-wake disorder* (N24SWD) and *irregular sleep-wake rhythm disorder* (ISWRD). N24SWD shows a pattern of sleep and wake which appears unassociated with the sun/moon light/dark cycle: it suggests that neither light nor social phenomena play a role in the sleep phase. The length of sleep is usually normal but the sleep phase seems to march forward based on the patient's intrinsic circadian rhythm (see **Figure 4D, 1–4,** page 180).

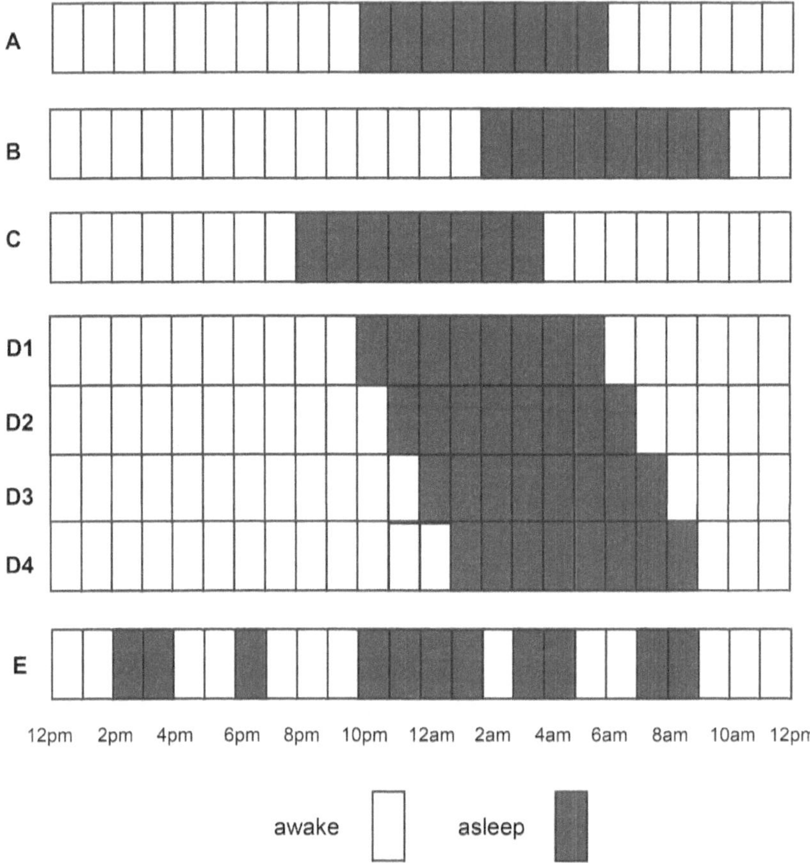

FIGURE 4. Circadian rhythm disorders. Sleep physicians frequently ask patients to keep sleep diaries and use these to create "sleep logs" that form a visual representation of the sleep pattern of each disorder. The above represent somewhat simplified examples of such logs. **A.** Normal sleep for a person who goes to sleep at 10pm and wakes at 6am, for a total sleep time of eight hours. **B.** A person who does not reverse the normal delayed sleep phase of adolescence on reaching their late teens or 20s and now has delayed sleep phase syndrome. This person cannot go to sleep before 2am and sleeps normally in quantity and quality (if allowed) until 10am. **C.** An older person with advanced sleep phase syndrome. This person finds it difficult to stay awake beyond 8pm and to stay asleep later than 4am. Sleep is usually punctuated by numerous arousals (not shown), which appear to be part of the aging process. **D1–4.** Four consecutive nights for a person with non-24-hour sleep-wake disorder, most commonly found in the visually impaired. This person's sleep phase shifts to a later time each night (usually by a few minutes, not hours). **E.** A child with irregular sleep-wake rhythm disorder. Sleep and wake are distributed over each 24-hour period with no discernable or repeatable pattern, only a chaotic one.

Bryan, a 38-year-old writer, had been almost completely blind since a fireworks accident in his teenage years. Since then he seemed always to have problems with daytime sleepiness and nighttime insomnia, but admitted that this pattern seemed to come and go; occasionally he was awake all day and slept well at night for a while.

I asked him to fill out, with help, sleep diaries for four weeks, denoting when he would go to bed, go to sleep, wake up, and rise from bed each morning. The diary showed an interesting pattern of gradual advancement of his sleep phase (as in Figure 4D, 1–4, page 180). Over four weeks his sleep onset advanced progressively from 10pm on the first night to 2:20am on the 28th night, which is an average of 10 minutes added to his sleep onset time each night.

He was diagnosed with non-24-hour sleep-wake disorder (N24SWD) and responded well to melatonin treatment.

The diaries suggested that Bryan's personal circadian rhythm was 24:10 (which is average), meaning that he was normally delayed by 10 minutes every night, as most of us are. But since he lacked the ability to be "reset" each morning by bright light, as his eyes did not transmit light impulses to his suprachiasmatic nucleus, he would fail to reset, or undo, his 10-minute delay each night. Instead his sleep became later by 10 minutes each night. After four weeks of this he found himself four hours and 20 minutes behind, as reflected in his sleep diaries.

As this progressed, his accumulated delay eventually resulted in a bedtime in the middle of the day and being awake all night.* He had no difficulty with sleep length. This pattern is called "free-running" sleep because the sleep phase adjusts forward each 24-plus hours unaltered by any zeitgebers ("time resetters"), apparently free of the influences of light or melatonin that normal people respond to.

---

* If his sleep time is advanced by 10 minutes nightly, that means it will be advanced by 12 hours every 72 nights (10 minutes × 72 = 720 min or 12 hours), so within 10 weeks he will be going to bed at noon rather than midnight, and then reverse again 10 weeks later.

Non-24 gives us a fascinating window into the world of the visually impaired. Remember from Chapter One that light normally enters our eyes through our pupils and travels to the back of the eye, the retina, where it creates electrical impulses in the retinal nerve. Some of these impulses travel to the occipital lobe of the brain where visual images are constructed: this is how we "see" what the light reflects from in front of us. The occipital lobes use those impulses to construct a mental image of what we are seeing: that's what "vision" is.

But other impulses from the retina travel not to the occiput but to the suprachiasmatic nucleus (the SCN) and promote the brain's intrinsic circadian rhythm (CR). If the average normal CR is 24 hours and 10 minutes (24:10) and the eyes are exposed to light every morning at about the same time, the brain will reset the CR back to 24 hours and *no* minutes and sleepiness will occur at about the same time every night— there will be no CR "drift." That extra 10 minutes is discarded.

For those with partial blindness, still able to perceive light and perhaps some blurry images, light effects on the retina are usually normal and CR is not affected. These are "blind" people who may sleep normally.

But as I explained to Bryan, above, in some totally blind people, if there has been extensive destruction of the retinas from disease, no light images come to the brain and they perceive only darkness; also, no retinal impulses make it to the suprachiasmatic nucleus (SCN) for the same reason, so the SCN gets no information to allow a reset of the circadian rhythm. The CR will drift, or "free-run," so the sleep phase becomes later each night. They find themselves unacceptably sleepy at times during the day and unacceptably awake at times during the night. This is true N24SWD.

Other totally blind persons who likewise have no visual images, who perceive only darkness, will still have normal CR, normal sleep-wake cycles, as long as they have normal resetting each morning as the rest of us do. This group may have eye disease severe enough to produce "total blindness" but not to a degree that has destroyed those special retinal cells that communicate with the SCN. This leaves the normal CR unaltered, and these people sleep and wake at normal times, being reset each morning by light with the rest of us—even though they may not perceive the light as "light". It appears that about half of blind persons are in this group, with normal CR; the rest have classic N24SWD, with drifting sleep-wake times.

Remember the three main resetting influences on CR? Light is the strongest, then melatonin, then social activities. If light is no longer a factor (because of eye disease), then the next best resetter is melatonin, and in fact melatonin treatment has been very successful in allowing blind persons to keep their sleep-wake cycle in sync with the rest of the world. Taking a low dose of melatonin at the same time every evening may be all that is needed to convert a non-24-hour situation to a precisely 24-hour one.

Irregular sleep-wake rhythm disorder (ISWRD) is the last of the five basic circadian rhythm disorders. It is also the most rare. An analysis of the sleep logs in this disorder (see **Figure 4E,** page 180) frustrates any attempt to find a repeatable pattern; the sleep phase is not just delayed or advanced, as in DSPS or ASPS, but broken up into pieces, sometimes up to four hours long, but in no predictable order. Instead, the sleep is distributed across the 24-hour period in a different pattern every day.

This is a problem found particularly in children with developmental disorders and in older patients with neurodegenerative disease, like Alzheimer's and Parkinson's disease, where abnormalities in the SCN are thought to be part of those diseases. You can imagine how difficult this might be to treat,[64] since the SCN itself has problems and may not respond well to extra light or melatonin.

PEARLS OF WISDOM

Circadian rhythm disorders are more common than previously thought. All persons who struggle to sleep at appropriate times should be screened by a sleep physician for these problems—especially young persons with difficulty awakening, visually impaired patients with sleeping issues, and older adults struggling to sleep. In many cases behavioral changes, light, and melatonin treatment can be very helpful.

Restless legs syndrome

Jerry was a 46-year-old plumber who had been healthy for most of his life. Over the previous year he began noticing "weird" sensations in his legs, mostly below the knees, when he would lie down to go to sleep at night. He found these difficult to describe to his wife or family, or to his doctor. Sometimes he could only say his legs felt like he had to move them, and in fact movement would help, at least temporarily.

Some evenings his legs would become uncomfortable when he sat down to watch TV after 9pm; at other times, his problems did not start until he retired to bed. He might improve by moving his legs around in bed but sometimes he found himself getting up to stretch and to walk around the bedroom to suppress the symptoms. Either way, he had difficulty falling asleep, sometimes for more than an hour, almost every night.

His primary care doctor diagnosed Jerry's problem as restless legs syndrome, and started him on a low dose of ropinirole, one pill at bedtime. This did not help at first, as his symptoms started a few minutes after taking the drug. Then Jerry tried taking it an hour before bed, and it helped a lot: he was able to fall asleep easily without leg symptoms.

After a successful six months he began waking around 3am a few times a week with those familiar leg symptoms and having difficulty going back to sleep. He doubled his dose, with some success, but more breakthrough symptoms a few weeks later prompted another doubling of his dose. Now things seem to be worsening: the "weird" sensations in his legs now began occurring earlier in the evenings and even in the afternoons, particularly when he was sitting down. He found it difficult to sit still for more than a few minutes at a time.

When he reported this to his physician, he was told that he had exceeded the maximum daily allowable dose for ropinirole, and that he may be experiencing "augmentation," a worsening of the problem caused by the medicine itself. He was referred to a sleep medicine physician, Dr. S., who checked Jerry's iron levels and found them to be normal. He confirmed augmentation and reassured Jerry that he would improve. He asked Jerry to stop ropinirole and switch to another drug (an "alpha-delta drug"). He warned him to expect some bad nights with unavoidable leg symptoms during the changeover.

This indeed occurred, but Jerry weathered through the difficult nights and now is doing well on his new drug. A test for venous disease in his legs was negative.

There are two words that are important in understanding restless legs syndrome: "syndrome" and "indescribable."

Restless legs syndrome, commonly known as RLS, has been recognized as problem since the 1600s. It is a *syndrome* because no one understands it very well—so it hasn't earned a disease name of its own. *Stedman's Medical Dictionary* defines a "syndrome" as "the aggregate of signs and symptoms associated with any morbid process, and constituting together the picture of the disease." The implication of this definition is that a syndrome is something that is so poorly understood that we can best describe it with a *picture* of it, namely a list of how it shows itself, rather than a name that explains the basic problem.

For example, an uncontrolled growth of white blood cells in the bloodstream might be called "high white blood cell count syndrome" if nothing else was known about it, but instead it's called "leukemia" which is more precise, a word that translates to "high white blood cell count" but carries the implication of cancer, its root cause. RLS does not have a root cause understood—yet—so it's just known by the sum of its symptoms, which are: an "indescribable" sensation in the legs that results in the urge to move them, a worsening of this feeling in the evenings and at rest, and improved symptoms on movement.

My ancient (1966) edition of *Stedman's Medical Dictionary*[65] defines RLS as "jimmy legs; jitter legs; a sense of indescribable uneasiness, twitching, or restlessness in the legs… caused by inadequate circulation… most common in neurotic patients." Thirty-three years later, the 1999 edition[66] of that dictionary no longer lists funny nicknames like "jimmy legs" and no longer suggests the patients are neurotic, still mentions "inadequate circulation," and mentions that antipsychotic medication might be involved.

Then 24 years later, the 2023 *Stedman's*[67] says RLS is "a sense of indescribable uneasiness, twitching, or restlessness that occurs in the legs after going to bed, frequently resulting in insomnia…thought to be caused by inadequate circulation or as a side effect of some SSRIs or other psychotropic medication."

Countless times in history various patients who were told their particular illness was due to neurosis or anxiety or depression were later diagnosed with a physical illness, sometimes leading to improvement or cure, once more was learned about the illness. It is an unfortunate feature of human nature to ascribe hard-to-explain complaints, like pain or numbness or dizziness, to some mental inadequacy of the patient—in essence, the doctor is saying, "Well, I can't explain this, so it must be the patient's weakness, instability or fault."

But it may not be the patient's fault at all, just an example of the physician's inadequate medical knowledge.

The lessons for the physician? Always reserve judgment on things you don't understand; you may understand them a lot better in the future, if you keep your mind and eyes open. Don't blame the patient for your (and the world's) inadequate knowledge about this problem.

The lessons for the patient? Sometimes unusual illnesses with unusual sensations have a physical cause; don't hesitate to get a second opinion if you're unsure. But some symptoms really are manifestations of anxiety or depression, so an open mind is still important.

Now RLS is defined in the Merriam-Webster online dictionary (February 2026) as: "a nervous disorder characterized by aching, crawling, or creeping sensations of the legs that occur especially at night usually when lying down (as before sleep) and cause a compelling urge to move the legs." We still consider RLS a "syndrome" because we cannot explain it much better in 2026 than in the last century, though we do have some clues.

One of those clues is the word "indescribable," which many patients themselves use in trying to communicate what they feel. They might say, "I have this *indescribable feeling* in my legs in the evenings when I lie down, and it drives me crazy. I have to move my legs around in bed or get up and walk around to make the feeling go away, which sometimes it does, and at other times just comes back again when I try to sleep. It usually doesn't bother me in the mornings or early afternoons."

Some people say the leg sensations feel crawly or tingly or pulling, and some say they are truly uncomfortable, throbbing, or even painful. Occasionally the discomfort involves the arms and even the trunk. When it's really severe, it can occur earlier and earlier during the day and throughout the night. No wonder some of these unfortunate patients in the past were considered neurotic! I'm sure they drove their physicians crazy with their unending complaints, unarmed as those physicians were with any real knowledge of the disease process or how to treat it.

We are a bit better on those fronts now. We don't know exactly what causes RLS, but we have gathered more details about it and some quite effective ways to treat it. Some progress has been made. Maybe one day RLS will graduate from being a syndrome, and even earn a real name!

It's a perplexing problem but here are a few things we've learned: It seems to have a circadian pattern: symptoms usually start in the evenings, then in some cases later recur during the night or earlier in the afternoons or even mornings when it's severe. It qualifies also as a "movement disorder," like Parkinson's for example (where muscle tremors are common) and is related to lower dopamine levels in the brain; medications that increase those levels can improve RLS. (But RLS is *not* a form of Parkinson's and does *not* lead to Parkinson's.)

RLS is also more common in people with anemia, especially iron-deficiency anemia, and iron replacement (either by mouth or intravenously) can produce dramatic improvement in a few patients. It is seen more often in patients with chronic kidney disease on dialysis or pregnancy (where anemia is more common) and in patients with neuropathy (where it isn't).

Depending on its severity, RLS can be only an occasional inconvenience, or it may be annoying, or more bothersome, or completely disruptive to a normal life and sleep. It is described as a "movement disorder" since it involves problems with muscle movement and occurs during wakefulness, but it is also considered a "sleep disorder" as it can prevent sleep onset and sleep maintenance for many people, and as it appears to have a circadian component, tending to start in the evenings and on lying down, and also because it can cause insomnia in other times of the night, waking people up during sleep and keeping them from falling back asleep.

Those fortunate patients with very mild RLS may need only the occasional leg massage or hot bath, or just movement of the legs briefly in or out of the bed. I myself have had rare "weird" feelings in my legs below the knees lying down in the evenings, maybe five times in the last 10 years, lasting maybe 15 minutes or less. I had that bizarre sense that I needed to move my legs and indeed they felt better when I did. I was lucky that the sensations did not recur. If indeed this was RLS, it was very mild. Lucky me.

Every patient with bothersome RLS should have iron levels tested. Iron metabolism plays a role in RLS, particularly iron metabolism in the movement areas of the brain. Finding low blood iron levels may justify iron replacement therapy in some of these patients; this can help symptoms, in some cases dramatically. That said, the actual role of iron in this context is not well understood.

The role of dopamine in RLS has proved to be one key to its treatment. As in Parkinson's, which is a more severe movement disorder, dopamine levels in the movement center of the brain in RLS are too low, and symptoms improve when dopamine levels are raised. Treatment of RLS involves some of the same drugs as for Parkinson's, but just lower doses.

Drugs like *ropinirole* and *pramipexole* are given as pills an hour or so before bedtime, so that there will be time for the blood level of the drug to rise before the patients lies down to go to sleep—which is commonly when symptoms start. These dopamine-raising ("dopaminergic") drugs (DAs) used to be first-line therapy for RLS, as they work so well initially, but they have developed a bad reputation recently because they predispose to a problem called "augmentation."[68]

Augmentation means that the symptoms have moved, both in time (to earlier and earlier times of the day) and in geography (from the legs to the arms and even the body), and is related to using higher doses of dopaminergic drugs. The unfortunate patient who "falls down the rabbit hole" with augmentation may have a very hard time working their way out, as weaning from the first drug and slow substitution of another (non-dopaminergic) drug will probably be necessary, and a number of bad nights with lots of symptoms may ensue.

It is estimated that some 50% of all patients treated with these drugs will develop augmentation. That is a big problem, since the medicines work so well at first, and so quickly, for most people. We've learned that higher doses promote augmentation, so we try to keep the dose as low as possible for as long as possible. It's not clear if gradual increases in the drug at times, as in Jerry's case above, pushes patients down that slippery slope toward augmentation, or if augmentation is more likely to occur on its own and higher drug doses are taken as a result.

Either way, holding a firm line on the doses, keeping a firm maximum daily dose that can never be exceeded appears to forestall augmentation, for a while at least. Interestingly, DAs can also cause impulsive behavior (like gambling or sexual activity) in a few people; it's important to be aware that this infrequent effect may be blamed on a drug.

Because of the issue of augmentation, other drugs have risen to the top of the preferred list, particularly the "alpha2-delta" drugs, such as *gabapentin* and *pregabalin*. Indeed, these are now considered the first choice for RLS. They can be a very effective treatment for RLS and importantly do not cause augmentation. They work through a protein called "alpha2-delta," which can block non-dopamine neurotransmitter output, and slow nerve transmission. They don't work as quickly as DAs but are considered safer. They do make some people sleepy, and more rarely, can cause confusion or breathing problems. They should not be taken with opiates.

Speaking of *opiates*, they have been recommended in the past for patients whose RLS is more "painful" than "indescribable." Opiates may be the best choice for this small percentage of RLS patients, particularly long-acting ones like methadone. However, understanding the increased concern over any but the shortest use of opiates in our society, given the potential for opiate addiction, taking great care is necessary in choosing the patients eligible for this approach.

Benzodiazepines, such as clonazepam, have been used with some success for RLS, but they are not as effective for most people as the other drugs above and do have drawbacks such as tolerance and habituation (more on this later).

Should everyone with RLS be tested for venous insufficiency? That ancient definition of RLS, the one from 1966 quoted above, related RLS to "inadequate circulation." Venous insufficiency, a problem that can occur in the legs when the surface veins dilate and can't control the flow of blood in the legs in its normal uphill travel, may be referred to as "varicose veins." These may appear as unsightly veins on the surface of the legs, or may not be so obvious, but it can also cause sometimes vague discomfort in the legs.

A number of studies have found that some of the people who go to a venous center for evaluation have both RLS and venous disease when tested, and perhaps 30% have improvement in their RLS symptoms, some completely made better, when venous disease is treated. That's not everyone, but it's still a significant number.

My takeaway from this is that everyone with RLS should also be checked for venous disease, and if there is any doubt, should be tested in a venous center. In the occasional situation, it might result in avoidance of lifelong medication for RLS.

Periodic limb movements

Where RLS is a problem that disrupts sleep to the point of sleep deprivation, periodic limb movements of sleep (PLMs) are not such a problem—not for the patient, at least. PLMs involve a certain kind of repetitive leg movement during sleep, more of a "pulling up" or jerking at the knee rather than a kicking movement, less likely affecting the arms. They can occur at any time during the night in non-REM sleep, in bunches of movements, or maybe just a few times; in some they occur hundreds of times per night.

They are frequently seen in RLS patients (80% have them, more with more severe RLS. But PLMs are not the same as restless legs, which is mainly a problem during wakefulness. They are seen commonly in other disorders like obstructive sleep apnea, REM sleep behavior disorder, and narcolepsy. But the largest group that show them are healthy normals.

Periodic limb movements are diagnosed with a standard sleep study when electrodes placed near the shins register leg movements, particularly if these movements are associated with arousals from sleep. Since most people who have sleep studies have some sort of complaint about their sleep, such as daytime sleepiness or frequent awakenings, for years it was thought that the PLMs in the sleep studies could cause those problems. Before the early 2000s, it was accepted practice to treat such movements, either with a benzodiazepine like clonazepam or a dopaminergic drug (DAs) like Sinemet (a precursor of ropinirole and pramipexole), and in many cases, patients seemed to improve.

But we may have been fooling ourselves. In 2005 when The American Academy of Sleep Medicine stated in its coding manual that "…PLMS with symptomatic sleep disruption is thought to be rare. The sleep of the bed partner is often more affected than that of the patient.[69] In other words, most people with PLMs don't have a problem from them alone, and treatment is not warranted.

The bedpartner, on the other hand, may well be bothered by their partner's leg jerks, so the treatment most recommended after that was…a bigger mattress. Keeping the sleeper apart from his or her bedpartner seems the most logical way to treat this problem. And this seems to work.

After 2005 we weaned lots of patients off the medicines they had taken (sometimes for years), for PLMs, and most did very well, not missing the medicines at all, reassuring us that that approach was right. The arousals we saw on sleep studies appear not to affect sleep quality.

Since that sea change in attitude about PLMs in 2005, more research into the significance of these movements have suggested some relationship to elevated blood pressure and to cardiovascular disease, including stroke and transient ischemic attacks, which may be related to too much sympathetic stimulation and systemic inflammation.[70] It's unclear what causes what; correlation does not prove causation.

There is not yet enough understanding of these relationships to justify any treatment to suppress the movements themselves; they may just be a manifestation of some third, unknown problem.

Certainly there is not enough evidence now to suggest that we treat these movements in an attempt to lower the risks of cardiovascular disease; more likely, PLMs may be a "para-phenomenon," a side issue of a larger (or not-so-large) problem, and not much of a problem in and of itself.

If you have PLMs, don't worry about them. Make sure you've had a checkup for heart and vascular problems, and…stay tuned.

PEARLS OF WISDOM

Restless legs syndrome can be mild or it can be devastating. Treatment options have been improving and, in fact, evolving rapidly, so the help of a sleep physician may be critical. Periodic limb movements may be harmless but the understanding of this problem is also in evolution.

CHAPTER 5

Not Sleepy Enough

Insomnia

Insomnia in general is the most common potential sleep problem facing humans. All of us at one time or another have problems with falling asleep when we want to, or staying asleep as late as we wish. If we're lucky, the problem is brief, lasting maybe a few nights at most, frequently related to some event in our lives (a relationship conflict, a stressful upcoming exam or social or work event, and so forth) that resolves on its own.

What we call *chronic insomnia* is the version that we as sleep medicine doctors see most in clinic, defined as a problem going to sleep and/or staying asleep at least three times a week for at least three months. It is associated with some emotional and/or physical consequences, such as fatigue, mood or memory problems, and daytime sleepiness and even accidents. Maybe one person in 10 has insomnia at this level.

Sometimes the answer to chronic insomnia is easy and straightforward, as simple as drinking less coffee and adjusting sleep habits. Sometimes the answer is elusive, as when one of a number of medicines the patient is taking has a subtle effect on their sleep. And sometimes the answer is difficult, as in dealing with severe anxiety or depression, or dealing with dependence on sleeping pills when the pills themselves no longer have the ability to induce sleep.

An initial evaluation of a person with insomnia involves a lot of questions; in fact, we worry about "questionnaire fatigue," as there are so many questions to ask that some people struggle to get through them all on the questionnaire. This is a difficult problem, as asking all those questions face-to-face invariably takes a lot longer, using a lot of time on the responses to some of the questions, responses that are really not helpful in the diagnosis and treatment; paradoxically, this can result in the patient having to return at a later date to complete the questioning, which delays any approach to treatment—much to the patient's frustration.

Best to complete the questionnaire at the beginning.

The questionnaire asks the patient about their routine bedtime, rise time, how long it usually takes to fall asleep, how often they wake during the night and for how long, how much coffee or tea they drink and when, what medicines they take and when, how they feel during the day, what their family history of sleep problems are, and so on.

Just as important as all these questions about insomnia are additional questions about other sleep disorders, especially obstructive sleep apnea (and, to a lesser extent, restless legs syndrome and circadian rhythm disorders). Not infrequently an underlying problem with subtle sleep apnea can result in difficulty maintaining sleep, a form of insomnia that will not improve until the breathing issue of sleep apnea is addressed.

Perhaps the most important part of the questioning is the exploration for possible anxiety or depression. At least 40% of all insomnia patients have sleep issues worsened by one or both of these problems; insomnia may not improve unless these issues are addressed. One question that may be a giveaway is "Do you think your sleep is problem is worsened by anxiety or depression?" Usually—but not always—the patient will answer "Yes," leading you right to the root causes of the problem.

Physicians constantly remind themselves that insomnia is a *symptom*. Physicians speak of "signs and symptoms" of a disease: the *signs* of something are those things that someone else (usually the physician) can *observe*: enlargement of the liver may be a sign of chronic alcohol use (detected on physical exam); the presence of changes in the optic nerve seen on exam may be a sign of glaucoma. The patient will not know of these "signs" until told by the physician. *Symptoms*, on the other hand, are *felt by the patient*: numbness and pain are symptoms of neuropathy; visual loss is a symptom of glaucoma. Symptoms are things described to the physician by the patient.*

We can think of insomnia as a *symptom* of something else: the patient describes the symptom of insomnia to the physician who considers that it is probably part of a larger problem. Lying awake for hours after our usual bedtime may be caused by drinking coffee in the evening; any list of side effects of caffeine will list "difficulty sleeping" as a common symptom. Difficulty sleeping is a symptom of the disorder we could call "caffeine overuse." Or: insomnia is a symptom of too much coffee.

Anxiety involves excessive worry and concern, and may cause such symptoms as fear, dread, restlessness, sweating, and rapid heartbeat; these are all symptoms of anxiety, and insomnia is another. (Importantly, night after night of difficulty sleeping can cause anxiety—fear of failure to perform, to fall asleep or to stay asleep—so anxiety can be a symptom of insomnia. Usually both must be addressed. This qualifies as *bidirectional*.

In general, if insomnia is a symptom of another problem, we must then find that other problem and deal with it before insomnia can improve. We could take a shortcut and jump right into insomnia treatment, but this is usually a formula for failure; it may miss the opportunity to find the root cause of the problem.

---

* This illustrates the error in logic made by the pharmaceutical industry in their efforts to market opioids in the last few years. They promoted the concept of pain being the "fifth vital sign" (the traditional four vital signs ["signs of life"] being temperature, heart rate, respiratory rate, and blood pressure). If a sign is something the physician detects and not something the patient feels, then "pain" cannot be a sign. And it isn't; it is clearly a symptom. This may have been an effective marketing technique, but it is incorrect and misleading.

Mary, 38, was a public relations officer for a large corporation. Her nine-year marriage to an attorney ended two years ago in a contentious divorce which left her anxious (worried and fearful about new relationships), reminiscent of problems with anxiety she had experienced in college. After her divorce she gained weight, and her young children began telling her that she was snoring.

She developed difficulty falling asleep and frequent awakenings at 4am daily, leaving her tired all day. More and more coffee helped less and less; it made her more anxious at work and made her insomnia worse. She tried making herself stay up later, to force herself to be sleepy so she could fall asleep, but this only increased her anxiety about sleeping and made her more tired during the day.

She saw her primary care physician who told her to cut back on coffee and gave her Ambien to take nightly. Initially she improved, but after a few weeks found that her insomnia returned and her usual dose of Ambien became less effective. She doubled, then tripled the dose; with each increase in dose, her sleep improved for a few nights, then worsened.

By the time she saw a sleep physician, she felt she was sleeping only two to three hours a night, was exhausted and anxious all the time, and fearful of running out of her Ambien. Her primary care physician tried switching her to another sleeping pill (trazodone) but she had even less success with this. She returned to Ambien.

A visit to a sleep physician resulted in a sleep study to exclude sleep apnea (she did not have it) and advice to taper coffee further and Ambien slowly. He sent her to a sleep psychologist who helped her explore her reactions to her difficult divorce and began a program of cognitive behavioral therapy for insomnia (CBTi) and for anxiety, along with a structured tapering schedule for Ambien, with eventual cessation.

One year after first starting Ambien, she was off all sleeping pills and sleeping well. She could fall asleep within 10 to 15 minutes of turning off her light, and averaged 7.5 hours of sleep, feeling more rested on awakening.

She did well for two years, but then her ex-husband, previously uninvolved, sued her for joint custody of her children. Again she experienced difficulty falling asleep and had early morning awakenings, waking suddenly at 4am or so frightened that she would lose her children. She reviewed some of the things she had learned in CBTi previously, and restarted practicing the concepts, which helped; she began to sleep normally again once her legal case was settled in her favor (and her ex-husband moved out of state).

In the example above, we could reason that Mary's insomnia was a *symptom* of the anxiety and depression she experienced as a result of her divorce. Until the basic cause—her anxiety—was addressed, it was less likely that her insomnia could resolve.

In dissecting out what promotes insomnia, we think of three categories of causes: predisposing, precipitating, and perpetuating causes. *Predisposing* causes are those in the background, those problems from the patient's past that can flare up under the right circumstances and cause new problems. In Mary's case, her history of anxiety in college reflected a tendency that could be reactivated again in the right circumstances. A diligent search of predisposing causes may find familial connections, and in Mary's case her mother had also been diagnosed with anxiety.

Anxiety in Mary's past predisposed her to insomnia later, given the right *precipitating* event, which in this case was the divorce (on top of, we might infer, the stresses of single motherhood combined with full-time work). So in the right *setting* (a person with this genetic background), a *triggering event* can set off or *precipitate* recurrence of those tendencies, and therefore insomnia. Treatment of both the insomnia and of the "emotional dysregulation"—the poor control of emotions that comes out as anxiety—must be considered to address the whole problem.

Once insomnia is treated and is improving, the patient may remain vulnerable to future triggering (precipitating) events; this happened to Mary, who was "re-triggered" into insomnia again when she was sued by her husband. Fortunately, the skills she had acquired in CBTi allowed her to overcome this setback without needing new formal medical care.

Frank, 24, was an intern for an architectural firm. The work was hard and demanded long hours, but he was generally in bed by 11pm most nights and slept to 7am, feeling well and alert in the mornings and throughout the day. During the recent recession, his firm downsized and he was let go. This was devastating for him, and with the sense of loss of self-worth unemployment can bring, and with the worry about finding another job, he began sleeping less at night—maybe five hours or so—making him feel more fatigued during the day. This made a new job search all the harder; he feared that his persistent weariness affected first impressions of him during interviews.

Determined to get more sleep, he started going to bed earlier and earlier, as early as 9pm, reasoning that he would then have more time to get more sleep. It didn't work. He found that this approach just gave him even more time in bed at night to stare at the ceiling and try to sleep—more time awake in bed, rather than more sleep. He became more frustrated and tired.

Good news came a few weeks later when a friend told him of another firm looking for an architect, and he was hired. The work was good and the pay even better than before. His worry lifted, but his insomnia persisted. Still going to bed at 9pm and getting up at 7am (10 hours in bed), he could not sleep more than five to six hours a night—though he no longer felt that worry about his job was keeping him awake.

A sleep physician recommended that he take a different approach, restricting rather than increasing his time in bed. At first he was asked to stay up until 1am each night, still getting up at 7am (six hours in bed), and continue this until he could sleep most of that time. He was not allowed to nap during the day. After a few nights of sleep restriction, he found he could fall asleep quickly at 1am and sleep until 7am.

His sleep physician then allowed him to go to bed an hour earlier, at midnight, and again after a week at this schedule he began sleeping most of the time he was in bed. When later he was allowed to begin going to bed at 11pm, he found he was back to the baseline where he had been before the job change: going to bed at 11pm, getting up at 7am, sleeping almost eight hours a night, and feeling quite well.

In Frank's story we are not given evidence of any *predisposing* causes of insomnia (a careful history might reveal some); clearly his job loss was the *precipitating* cause, the event that tipped him over from a good sleeper to a not-so-good one. What this story does illustrate well is the concept of *a perpetuating* cause of insomnia; as many people with insomnia do, Frank reasoned that spending more time in bed might give him more time to grab random bits of sleep, with an overall result of more total sleep, but instead, this made things worse.

Even though his precipitating cause (unemployment) had been removed, when he got a new and better job, his insomnia persisted as it was perpetuated by his bad sleep habits. Spending more time in bed, rather than increasing total sleep, seems to increase "performance anxiety" of not being able to sleep, as there are more hours spent lying awake than before. Things get worse rather than better. When these habits were reversed with "sleep restriction therapy," his insomnia improved.

Billy, 37, worked in financial services. His job was demanding and his work hours were long. He sometimes had difficulty staying asleep, waking at 4am and having difficulty falling back to sleep— usually not going back to sleep at all. He felt sleepy during the day and had on rare occasions fallen asleep in front of his computer at work. He had gained a lot of weight in the past five years; he admitted to drinking two cocktails in the evenings with dinner. He was single, but had a girlfriend, Gail, who frequently stayed over.

He asked his primary care physician for help with insomnia, and was sent to a sleep physician, Dr S. Gail came with him to the evaluation.

Billy told Dr S. that his sleep problems, both the early-morning awakenings and the daytime sleepiness, had worsened in the past five years, and Gail noted that he had been snoring and occasionally gasping during sleep over that time. Dr S. did not feel that Billy had significant anxiety or depression to explain early awakenings, but did suspect obstructive sleep apnea.

A subsequent sleep study confirmed moderate obstructive apnea, and CPAP, weight loss, and tapering of alcohol were prescribed. His nighttime sleep and daytime sleepiness improved dramatically with CPAP, which he used faithfully. Sleeping pills were not used.

Two years later, he had lost significant weight and tried stopping CPAP; Gail said he no longer snored nor had gasping during sleep without CPAP now, and he continued to feel alert during the day. Dr S. ordered a home sleep study which showed that his sleep apnea had resolved. He officially stopped CPAP, and advised Billy that if he could avoid future weight gain and avoid most alcohol, he might continue to avoid a return of obstructive sleep apnea and any associated insomnia.

Because sleep apnea is so pervasive in modern society, it must be considered in any sleep evaluation. Whereas the stereotypical sleep apnea patient is an obese middle-aged male who snores, has witnessed apneas, and is excessively sleepy during the day, not everyone with sleep apnea fits that stereotype. Many do, but there are many others with significant sleep apnea who are very young, or old, or female, and/or thin, who aren't aware of snoring and have not been told of stopping breathing, snorting or gasping during sleep, and are not measurably sleepy during the day.

An open mind is important in finding sleep apnea, and a sleep study may be necessary to exclude it. In Billy's case, it was a little easier to suspect and to justify a sleep study, which proved the diagnosis. If insomnia were treated without considering the possibility of contributing problems—and this happens with some frequency—there is much less chance of re-establishing normal sleep and health.

Now let's look at a more serious problem. What do you think constitutes the ultimate professional failure in therapy for any physician? It has to be the supreme failure to improve or preserve health, which means…death. But not all death is failure; sometimes it's natural.

How that failure is perceived is entirely a matter of what treatments are available: if an oncologist is treating a patient with chemotherapy and the patient dies of their leukemia nonetheless, that is a failure of treatment. If the chemotherapy is the best treatment available at that time for that illness, and if the death occurs because of the severity of the leukemia, overwhelming whatever benefit the chemotherapy could offer, then we might judge that the patient's death is not the physician's "fault," as it appears there was nothing more that could be offered in that situation.

Does the oncologist still feel that she is a "failure" in that setting? Many will. It's human nature. Our sworn goal as physicians is to preserve health and prolong life. I myself have attended to dozens of patients who have died of various causes, most commonly from critical illnesses in the ICU, or of emphysema or other lung disease when I practiced pulmonology. In almost all of those cases every possible thing that was appropriate to do, or try to do, to preserve life was done or tried, but with poor outcomes.

Standing at their bedsides as they died, I could only wish that other treatments were available, or other more effective preventative measures (like smoking cessation) had been utilized earlier. Wishful thinking. This could still be considered a failure of the system, and a personal failure for me as a physician. Even worse: two of my patients (over a period of 50 years of practice) committed suicide related to unremitting lung disease, and I did not (nor did anyone else, in the medical community or in the patient's family) see this coming. It was a shock both times and produced in me a profound sense of failure.

What does all this have to do with sleep? Let's look at an example of the worst possible outcome of insomnia. This example is fictional, but it is based on a true story.

Marty, 58, was an interior decorator, a married mother of three. She saw a sleep physician, Dr B, at the request of her psychiatrist, who was treating her for depression and anxiety. She described a history of worsening insomnia, both sleep-onset insomnia and sleep-maintenance insomnia, over many years, and had had minimal improvement in sleep with antidepressants and multiple trials of different sleeping pills. She expressed the belief and hope that the next sleeping pill, the newest on the market perhaps, would be the one to solve her sleeping problem.

Her father had managed a grocery store when she was a child. When she was 11, and in the store with her father after hours, a man with a gun tried to rob the store. He tied up both her and her father in the back room of the store, and vowed to kill both of them after he had emptied the cash register. When he went to the front of the store to get the money, her father, despite being tied to a chair, managed to reach his own gun in a drawer, and when the man returned, shot him in full view of Marty. The robber survived and was subsequently sentenced to a long jail term.

Marty and her father, along with her mother and brother, buried this experience. As terrifying as it was, her parents decided it was best for the family that, once the trial and its notoriety were past, the unhappy circumstances would never be discussed again. The parents made a vow that this secret would remain in the family, and the children had to agree. Marty spent the rest of her life pretending that this event had not happened, and did not tell even her husband about this experience when she married in her mid-30's.

She began having difficulty sleeping in her 20s, and over the years was given various hypnotics (sleeping pills) by a number of primary care physicians. She did not tell them about her childhood experiences. After many years, she was referred to a psychiatrist, and the history of her childhood trauma emerged. The psychiatrist felt that her insomnia was a result of underlying anxiety and depression from that experience, the memory of which had festered in her mind for some decades. He was also concerned that she was addicted to hypnotics. He started antidepressants and asked her to see both a sleep psychologist and a sleep physician. Both of whom then learned her history of trauma.

The sleep psychologist started a program of cognitive behavioral therapy for insomnia (CBTi) and gradual tapering of her hypnotics, but Marty struggled with this as her insomnia worsened. On her first meeting with Dr B, the sleep physician, she tearfully recounted that she "had not slept in weeks" and did not know where to turn. Dr B evaluated her for other background sleep disorders that might contribute to insomnia but found none.

He urged her to continue with CBTi and visits with the psychiatrist and psychologist and offered her a new-to-the-market hypnotic. Dr B later learned that Marty's insurance company had denied coverage for the new hypnotic, which would have cost her $900 a month out-of-pocket. She did not buy it.

Three days after her last visit with him, Dr B received a call from the psychiatrist to report that Marty had committed suicide.

All of the professionals caring for Marty felt a sense of professional failure for her situation and wondered what else could have been done to prevent her death. Involuntary institutionalization is available for impending suicide, but only if there is reason to believe suicide is imminent; in Marty's case, no one suspected suicide as she had not described thoughts of self-harm to her family or anyone else, even when questioned.

Regular hospitalization for insomnia is not covered by insurance companies; psychiatric hospitalization for hypnotic addiction is occasionally allowed and might have been an option for her at some point when other attempts failed. CBTi was considered a good approach for her, but this process takes time. Her doctors were saddened and frustrated that it seemed that nothing could have been done to prevent Marty from taking her own life.

Marty's story indeed represents the worst possible outcome in the treatment of insomnia. Understanding as we do that insomnia is usually a symptom of something, in Marty's case we can see that her suicide was a failure in the treatment of anxiety and depression, a fact with which her fictional psychiatrist would undoubtedly agree. It was striking to hear that her brother, who had been told to keep secret the traumatic event that so affected Marty's life, continued to deny that event after her death.

We don't know if he believed what he said when he told the mourners at her funeral that she died of a sleep disorder or not, but sleep physicians would more likely attribute her suicide to her underlying anxiety and depression, which resulted in her insomnia, rather than to the insomnia itself. This is not to deny that insomnia can greatly exacerbate those problems.

Reviews in the medical literature[71] exploring the link between suicide and insomnia have struggled with precise definitions of insomnia and how much to attribute suicide to the sleeping issue, and how much to the underlying anxiety and depression.

Why is this important?

Because insomnia is almost always a symptom of something, and that something may be as important, if not more important, than the insomnia itself when treatment is considered. Understanding anxiety and depression can be critical in understanding the basis of insomnia.

Falling or not falling

Let's switch gears now and think about what it means to fall asleep. You may recall from earlier in this book (see page 21) that we humans normally cycle through three different forms of consciousness in each 24-hour period, which for simplicity we have named "wake," "non-REM sleep," and "REM sleep." Clearly we are most aware of our surroundings when we are awake; in fact, we think of wake as that state when our senses of smell, taste, touch, feel, and hearing are most acute, and most in contact with our immediate environment.

To be awake is to be *aware:* aware of the reality of the world around us, with all its attractions and threats. We start to lose our senses, our awareness, when we fall asleep; we become less able to hear or see anything around us, and once we're beyond stage N1 (shallow) sleep, we perceive much less from the outside.

Consider a torture situation (sorry): you are held in prison against your will, and a loud high-pitched pulsating tone is played in your cell all day and night. Sleep will be very difficult, if not impossible, no matter how sleep-deprived you are, and when it does occur, in fragments, it will not be helpful. What if, instead, a terrible smell is substituted for the sound? Again, terrible sleep, if any.

In fact, any situation in which you are subjected to any persistent, severe sensory stimulation will prevent sleep. Sleep requires disconnection from the environment, and if our environment insists on stimulating alarm systems in the brain, preventing disconnection from the outside, sleep may seem impossible.

So we must *disconnect* when we want to change our state of consciousness from wake to non-REM sleep (it's unusual to fall asleep directly into REM sleep, as we discussed in the chapter on narcolepsy, page 156). To get from W (wake) to N1 (stage 1 non-REM) sleep requires letting ourselves *fall away* from our sensory inputs, letting ourselves *fall asleep*.

I love that word "fall," as it so accurately transmits that sense that as we move into sleep, we experience a feeling of descent or free-fall from a mental high place as we leave one part of our world for another. We unplug our senses, removing ourselves from the environment that still wants to make its presence known through our ability to detect texture (our bed sheets), sounds, smells, and light in our bedroom. We divorce ourselves from these inputs, assisted by our various drives to, or hunger for, sleep—as we discussed in Chapter One.

It's important to understand that disconnection is an absolutely necessary requirement for sleep to occur, along with the concept that *sleep itself is defined by the act of disconnection*. We won't sleep unless we're disconnected, but being disconnected does not prove sleep: for example, no one mistakes an NFL player who is knocked unconscious on the field by a direct blow to the head as being asleep. Clearly, this player has a concussion and his disconnection from his environment comes from head trauma and—hopefully—only transient brain damage. This is not sleep.

Thus our logic allows us another way of looking at insomnia: it is a *failure to disconnect*. It is a failure to move from wake to non-REM sleep, because lack of disconnection means continued stimulation, which promotes continued wake. We know instinctively to make our sleeping environment as non-stimulating as possible so as to optimize the onset of sleep. We want a quiet, dark, cool, non-odorous bedroom and a comfortable mattress, sheets, and pillows; lacking any of these, sleep may be harder to achieve. We also consider our attempt for sleep should occur in the right phase of our circadian rhythm, which usually means after a normal amount of time spent awake after our previous sleep episode.

If all these elements are present, we have optimized our likelihood of falling asleep. If we still cannot transition into non-REM sleep after an appropriate amount of time (15 to 20 minutes or so), then we must ask: Is disconnection from the environment being blocked by continued stimulation?

In the absence of detectable physical stimulation (such as a high bedroom temperature, pain from a recent injury, and so forth), that stimulation must be non-physical, i.e., mental. At one time or another, we have all experienced racing thoughts at bedtime preventing sleep, disturbing thoughts which may arise from a recent argument, from difficulty with one's job or family or relationships during the day, or from many other causes in our mental, emotional and even spiritual lives.

If the emotional impact of these thoughts is mild, our drive to sleep will overcome this stimulus and we will fall asleep despite it. If the impact is severe, sleep may not be achievable at all, or we may eventually fall asleep after a long period of trying, and then, after some of our sleep drive has been satisfied by a few hours of sleep, we may awaken early—typically at 3–4am, when our normal circadian rhythm promotes a rise in potential alertness—and revisit these thoughts and emotions again. We can think of racing thoughts as an indicator of anxiety, and we can think of anxiety as a chemical state (yes, with increased stress hormones) that prevents disconnection, and thereby promotes insomnia.

The two main forms of insomnia, sleep initiation problems and sleep maintenance problems, happen to most of us at some point in our lives, and are usually transient, lasting only a night or two, and do not require treatment or medical intervention. This is "acute insomnia," a mild problem of short duration, and is differentiated from "chronic insomnia," which by definition lasts more than three months.

It is easy to see now why anxiety and depression are two of the biggest drivers of insomnia in humans. Both involve issues with disturbing thought patterns day and night; both involve worrisome thoughts that can block sleep by preventing disconnection from the environment by their ever-present mental stimulation. About half of all the patients who come to sleep doctors for help with insomnia are diagnosed with anxiety and/or depression, and as we have seen, trying to treat the symptom of insomnia alone (just treating the inability to sleep) without dealing with the underlying cause, the persistent stimulation, is far less likely to be successful.

Can we stop this bombardment of the brain by these intrusive thoughts by other means? What can we do to the brain to make it stop stimulating itself, to make it disconnect?

Patients with severe insomnia, so desperate as they are to achieve sleep, beg for anything that will give them sleep. What can we do for them? A blow to the head, as in our NFL player above, would produce unconsciousness, not sleep. An inhaled anesthetic, as given in the operating theater, would produce anesthesia, which also is not sleep.

Hypnotics (the name comes from *Hypnos*, the Greek god of sleep), also known as *sleeping pills,* might seem to be the answer, as people who take them do achieve something that looks like sleep on EEG (see Chapter One, page 31 about sleep stages), but there are arguments that "real" or "healthy" sleep is not achieved. We will look at these arguments later, in a detailed discussion of hypnotics. But, for now, it seems more logical to conclude that the best way to manage a failure of disconnection caused by continued mental stimulation from anxiety, depression, or other forms of intrusive thoughts is to deal directly with those thoughts.

One way to avoid these thoughts is with *quiet distraction.* We have all done this when we are bothered by something and can't sleep, or even when we don't know what bothers us, and we can't sleep. For example, you may have tried counting imaginary sheep in your mind, or mentally counting all the windows in your house, or (in my case) mentally listing the 50 American states in alphabetical order. These are all ways of forcing yourself to think of something other than the problem of falling asleep.

These mental exercises can work as long as they can truly distract— if the underlying intrusive thoughts can't intrude through the distraction—and they don't engender anxiety from failure to perform. If you obsess about how many windows there really are in one particular room or, again in my case, when I get upset that I can't remember "Idaho" when I'm going through the "I" section of the alphabet in the list of the states, then this distraction is not distracting enough. (Listing the states has rarely worked for me, for that reason.)

Distraction comes in other forms, such as using a noisemaker in the bedroom (my wife loves a low-pitched, continuous white noise, which distracts but also masks any other random noises at night), listening to low-volume music, podcasts, or even TV for some (though the light from the TV can be stimulating), and many other ways. Noisemakers now come in a number of "colors": white noise, pink noise, brown noise, and so forth, depending on the wavelengths of sound chosen. All may be worth trying.

As long as the distracting effect of the distraction is stronger than its stimulating effect, it may allow one to not hear intrusive thoughts and thus slip into sleep. It may not be clear whether a particular distracting or masking technique will work until it is tried.

Some years ago I joined 180 horseback riders on a trail ride in California. Camping outside at night, we slept on cots near an enormous truck-sized generator that provided all the camp's power. This gas-powered generator made a dramatically loud (I'm guessing 80 decibels or so), continuous, low-pitched noise all night, but everyone slept well near it. Remarkably, when the generator ran out of fuel in the middle of the night, the entire camp was awakened by the sudden *silence*, and, once the generator was refueled and fired up again, everyone quickly fell asleep again when the loud noise returned. This is an example of how *changes* in the auditory environment can also cause arousal from sleep.

When intrusive thoughts are too powerful to allow distraction, stronger efforts may be necessary. The next logical approach would seem to be sleeping pills; what could be simpler than popping a pill at bedtime and getting great sleep? Most people do not do well with the same sleeping pill nightly for very long.

But over the past few years I have seen a small number of patients who describe having taken the same hypnotic (usually Ambien) for more than a decade with the same satisfactory response: a good night's sleep. I always worried about these patients, wondering if I was somehow missing something in their histories that might explain their success with hypnotics that few others could achieve. The fact is that only a few people successfully use sleeping pills for a long time.

Let's look at why.

The hypnotic paradox

When I was in medical training in the 1970s, on occasion I was called into the Emergency Room to see someone with an acute barbiturate overdose. Barbiturates were the main class of sleeping pills then; they have all but disappeared from the market for treatment of insomnia since that time, though a few are still used for other things, such as anesthesia or seizure disorders. The old oral barbiturates had names like Seconal, Nembutal, and Amytal.

This class of drugs slows nerve cell transmission, and so produces sedation and a form of sleep. The problem is in the overdose: as we have seen, when insomnia accompanies anxiety and depression, the risk of suicide must be considered whenever treatment for insomnia is prescribed.

Fifty years ago, there was little that could be done to preserve life when a patient took a high dose of barbiturates in an attempt at suicide. Many of these patients died after a period of coma, despite having arrived alive at the hospital and having the proper diagnosis and treatment and having any residual barbiturate removed by stomach lavage. There was, and still is, no "reversal drug" for barbiturates. Treatment is "supportive," which means normal support of blood pressure, oxygenation, fluid balance, nutrition, and…hope.

Hope did not save many of those lives.

Imagine, then, our delight when a new class of sedative-hypnotics came on the market: the benzodiazepines ("benzos"). Valium and Librium were two of the early new ones. These drugs were much safer than the barbiturates; when a patient with a suicide attempt from benzos arrived at the hospital, whether alert or sleepy or comatose, once it was clear that no other drugs were involved, they could just safely "sleep it off." And they did. They woke later with little physical or mental damage. It's just harder to commit suicide with benzos.

Not surprisingly, benzos then became popular drugs for the treatment of insomnia. Numerous new versions of this group were developed, some with more sedative properties, some more anti-anxiety, some shorter acting, some longer.

Two important relatives ("cousins") of benzos acted similarly but were not truly benzos; instead, they "act like" benzos in that they attach to the same receptor sites on the nerve cell to produce similar effects, so they are called "receptor-agonists," and they tend to be lumped in the broad category of "benzodiazepines." I mention this because these two are some of the most commonly prescribed drugs of all kinds *in the world*, and their names are Ambien (zolpidem) and Lunesta (eszopiclone). It's likely you have heard of them.

Benzos are not the only hypnotics on the market now, but they are still an important category. Some of the other categories of medications used to induce sleep are antihistamines, antidepressants, antipsychotics, melatonin, and orexin blockers.

Let's concentrate on the benzos first.

In the medical community we felt safe in prescribing benzodiazepines for sleep in the last half of the 20th century, and even today, short-term use is considered safe and in many cases, effective. The key word in that last sentence is "short-term." Early on, most published studies looked only at short-term use of sleeping pills, to establish efficacy (did they increase sleep) and safety, as it's more expensive and more complicated to conduct drug studies that last longer than 30 days.

Most drug inserts (the official information from the manufacturer on the allowable and proper use of a drug) suggest safe use of a hypnotic for 30 days or so. But that may not be the way the drugs are used. If I need Ambien to sleep at night and it works throughout May, can't I continue to use it through June? July? Next year? If I like it, and it works, you may have difficulty getting me to stop using it. I may hound you, my physician, to keep prescribing it. That's a problem.

And it's just one of the problems that have emerged over the years as we have looked at sleeping pills in general, and benzos in particular. Other problems include the potential for addiction, tolerance, rebound insomnia, next-day impairment, increased accidents, cognitive problems, and possibly increased risk of dementia. Somewhat surprisingly, increases in infections and even cancer have been reported. These problems are discussed in detail below.

What is the difference between habituation and addiction? If I say I am addicted to eating peanut butter crackers in the evenings, I may be saying that I look forward to them at my usual time and will miss them if I can't have them. But I would be wrong to say I am addicted: to be precise, I am not addicted but rather *habituated* to peanut butter—because I do not go into "withdrawal" when I miss my crackers.

Addiction differs from habituation in that there is a *defined withdrawal syndrome* in addiction that occurs in the absence of the needed substance. A simple example is oxycontin, a highly addictive painkiller, withdrawal from which can cause fever, diarrhea, nausea, vomiting, anxiety, agitation, and many other symptoms. (I don't get any of these when I miss my PB crackers, just a wistful longing.)

We can name many addictive substances in our world: alcohol, nicotine, cocaine, opium, heroin, morphine, fentanyl, other opiates, and so on. All of these have defined withdrawal syndromes. This occurs with benzos as well, though apparently only after prolonged treatment.[72] Short-term treatment is safer in this regard; one is unlikely to become addicted to benzos after a few nights' use or a few weeks' use, but longer than that entails some risk. The safest course is to use them for no longer than the manufacturers' (and the researchers') recommendations: no more than 30 nights.

Is this doable? The answer is yes, particularly if during that time efforts have been made to change the circumstances—or the responses to those circumstances—causing the insomnia. If nothing has changed by the time the 30 nights have passed, it's less likely that insomnia will not just re-emerge in the absence of any hypnotic. Currently the best non-medical approach to alter the course of insomnia is cognitive behavioral therapy for insomnia (CBTi), to be discussed below.

Let's look at some of the problems that can occur with benzodiazepines when used long-term. Sleeping pills in other categories may have some or none of these problems (as well as some problems specific for that category); we will discuss these later.

Tolerance to a medication means that, over time, higher and higher doses are required to produce the same results. This is an important issue with benzos. A person with insomnia may find the need to increase the dose of their sleeping pill over time to continue to get the same effect. The recommended maximum dose for zolpidem (brand name Ambien) is 5 mg nightly for females and 10 mg for males, yet I have seen a number of patients, both male and female, taking much higher doses, and still struggling to sleep.

Robert, 34, was pleased to be an associate at a large New York law firm, but he worried that he was not moving up in the path to partner as effectively as he had hoped. He worked long hours and did not always get much sleep, but even when he was not working, he found that sleep was impeded by racing thoughts about his job status. His doctor gave him Ambien 10 mg "for occasional use," but over a year's time he increased usage from once or twice a week to nightly. For a while, he could fall asleep and stay asleep with this dose, but eventually he found himself waking at 4am most mornings despite Ambien. The resultant loss of sleep made his hardworking days all the more difficult, and he became more desperate for sleep.

He began adding a half pill to his dose, now 15 mg nightly, which helped only for a few months. Again he began struggling to get to sleep and stay asleep. He increased his dose again and again, ultimately reaching a dose of 30 mg nightly—three times the maximum-recommended dose for males. Once more this dose helped at first, then failed to give him sleep. He ran out of pills long before his refill was allowed, and he panicked. He called his doctor.

He was referred to a sleep physician, who added another hypnotic to his regimen while beginning a gradual taper of the Ambien, and brought in a sleep psychologist for cognitive behavioral therapy for insomnia (CBTi). His insomnia improved slowly; there were many difficult nights but eventually he was able to stop all hypnotics, to come to grips with the stresses of his job, and to sleep well without pills.

Like Robert above, some patients on benzodiazepines slowly increase their doses over months to years, with each increase achieving better sleep for a while, but then, as more tolerance develops, losing that benefit and needing to increase the dose again. Eventually the drug becomes useless for sleep, but stopping causes severe withdrawal, with worsening insomnia. These unfortunate patients require an aggressive approach to insomnia treatment, usually CBTi combined with a slow, gradual tapering of the zolpidem and usually transient substitution of another drug to limit withdrawal. In severe cases of addiction with tolerance at this level, in-patient treatment of withdrawal symptoms may be necessary, possibly in a psychiatric facility.

Rebound insomnia may occur whenever a hypnotic is stopped after prolonged use: the resultant insomnia recurs and is as severe, or worse, than before the drug was started. This is always a disappointment to the sleeper and may be a sole symptom of drug cessation or a part of an overall withdrawal syndrome. Rebound insomnia occurs frequently with benzos and is one of the main reasons that short-term use without other non-medical assistance, like CBTi, may fail. It is also a reason for patients to believe that they cannot ever sleep without medications again.

Increased accidents may be caused by any sedating drug, hypnotics included, when the dose is such that blood levels remain high during the day: this is called *next-day impairment.* There may be more falls and resultant fractures, and more automobile accidents, especially with the use of longer-acting drugs, which build up in the brain with continued use.

For example, clonazepam (Klonopin) is a benzo that is used for both insomnia and anxiety. It has a half-life of around 18 hours, which means that, if it is taken once a day, the amount in the bloodstream each morning is just under half of what it was the day before; adding a new dose each day results in a gradually increasing blood level over days and weeks that may lead to profoundly depressing effects on brain function.

Everyone is vulnerable to this effect, but again, the elderly are most at risk. An increase in falls translates to an increase in hip fractures, hospitalizations, surgeries, postoperative complications, and death. An increase in driving accidents adds to these risks.

Cognitive issues—difficulty with learning, concentration, memory (and episodes of amnesia), and judgment, even delirium—are potential side effects of all sedatives and hypnotics, especially the longer-acting ones, and also fall into the category of next-day impairment. Elderly and not-so-elderly people who have been suspected of early dementia based on worsening mental function are occasionally diagnosed instead with sedative or hypnotic overuse, and may make a complete recovery when the drugs are stopped.

Any evaluation of cognitive dysfunction must include a review of all medications, with sedating drugs most suspect. And of course, adding alcohol or other sedating medications to doses of sleeping pills risks significant nervous system depression...and even death.

Evidence suggests that *dementia* is a risk from long-term use of some hypnotics. This is a difficult risk to prove, however, and has been considered controversial until recently, when more information has become available, incriminating benzos more than other drugs.[73] Looking at multiple studies involving almost four million patients, the use of any hypnotic for more than 100 nights increased the risk of dementia by 5%. That's only a bit over three months' usage. And that's scary.

Because anxiety frequently accompanies dementia (anxiety over worsening memory loss, for example) and because benzos are frequently prescribed for anxiety, one could ask if the dementia that subsequently is diagnosed is not due to the drug, but was already in its earliest stages when the drug was prescribed. If the dementia onset preceded the prescription of a drug, the drug cannot be blamed for the dementia.

A number of large-scale studies of the relationship between benzos and dementia have tried to overcome this concern by requiring a minimum period of time (e.g., five years) between drug prescription and dementia diagnosis for that case to be counted, reasoning that "early dementia" should show itself before that time has elapsed—so the drug must be a contributor to the dementia. When these restrictions are in place, there is still an increased risk of dementia (Alzheimer's) in long-term users of benzos, more for the longer-acting than shorter-acting drugs.[74,75] Overall, the risk for dementia with use over 180 days for the average drug was increased by 50%; for the long-acting ones, like clonazepam (Klonopin), the increase was in the range of 75%.

Because of these and other side effects of benzodiazepines, there has been a call for their use to be restricted only to prescription by psychiatrists.[76] As of February 2026, this has not happened.

There are lots of other sleeping pills out there, some over-the-counter medications, some health-food supplements, some prescription drugs designated for other purposes but used to induce sleep, and some newer hypnotics designed specifically with modern understanding of the neuroscience of sleep.

Let's look at some of these.

Antihistamines have been used as sleeping pills for decades. These are available over the counter (OTC) and are easily recognized when a brand-name is attached to the suffix "PM." There are many examples, such as "Tylenol-PM," "Allergy-PM," etc. In each case a standard drug, like acetaminophen, is combined with an antihistamine like diphen-hydramine (Benadryl) or doxylamine.

We think of histamine as a chemical in the body that takes part in allergic reactions, but it is also a neurotransmitter that promotes *alertness* in the brain. Blocking it can cause sleepiness, which is how anti-histamines work as a sleeping pill. This applies more to first-generation antihistamines, like Benadryl; the later versions, like Claritin and Zyrtec, are better for allergy as they are less likely to cause sleepiness.

Antihistamines may be okay for occasional use but we rarely meet patients who successfully use them nightly, as they seem to lose their potency as sleeping pills (but still function well for allergies) after two to three nights. Cognitive problems—confusion, memory issues—in the elderly can occur with antihistamines, as well as falls, and dementia with long-term use may be a risk—but there is less evidence for this than for the benzodiazepines.

Some *antidepressants* and *antipsychotics* may be used "off-label" as sleeping pills if they happen to have sleepiness as a side effect, especially if there are underlying mental issues that could also be addressed by the drug. These drugs may have side effects other than the ones we discussed with benzodiazepines. Examples of antidepressants that also cause sleepiness are trazodone (Desyrel) and quetiapine (Seroquel), both of which may lower or block histamine. Both are used frequently for their sleep-inducing qualities, but they also have their own adverse reactions; both can cause cardiac arrhythmias and EKG changes.

Melatonin is potentially one of the safest ways to induce sleep. Recall that melatonin is a hormone from the pineal gland that signals the brain that it is time to go to sleep, and in humans, that signal is elicited by darkness. What we call low doses of melatonin—in the 0.5 to 1.0 mg range—are those that produce blood levels similar to normal

darkness-induced levels. We use such doses in circadian rhythm disorders (especially delayed sleep phase syndrome in young persons) to
nudge the onset of sleepiness toward a desired time. Higher doses of
melatonin (3–10mg) are more directly sleepiness-inducers—they actually make one sleepy.

Many people use melatonin nightly (and the press has reported, with
some concern, that a large number of children are being given melatonin now). Melatonin appears to be much safer than benzos: there may be
less tolerance, less next-day impairment (but still some daytime sleepiness), fewer falls and accidents, less likelihood of dementia. Remarkably,
melatonin may have some antioxidant and anti-inflammatory effects,
even some anticancer effects. Overall, it is quite safe.

Melatonin would appear to be a great choice for a sleeping medication, except for one thing: it is considered a *dietary supplement* by
the FDA, not a medication, and is therefore not regulated to the same
degree. Studies of various dietary supplements sold in chain outlets
have shown wide variability in how much of the target drug was actually
present (sometimes none, sometimes much more than the therapeutic
level) and in how much *else* was present (and not listed on the label),
with undesirable drugs and even plant and vegetable material sometimes evident.[77]

It is difficult to have confidence when taking most supplements as
medicines—note the standard disclaimer on their labels that states "This
product is not intended to diagnose, treat, cure, or prevent any disease."

So what *is* it intended to do, if not any of the things we usually take
medications for?

There are two ways to deal with this dilemma. The first is to screen
the labels of all supplements, including melatonin, for those that are
approved by the *United States Pharmacopeia* (USP), which means looking for "USP Verified" on the label. USP is a nonprofit organization
that tests ingredients in some supplements and compares them to their
labels. Approved drugs in various categories are listed on their website.
This gives us a bit more confidence that the medication on the label

is the medication we are actually taking—and not much else. You can check on their website for any supplement they have verified, but unfortunately, it's not all of them.

The second way to feel safe in using melatonin is to use a "receptor agonist" of melatonin, meaning using a drug that plugs into the same receptors in the brain as melatonin, and thereby produces similar effects. Ramelteon is one such drug. The good news is that it is approved by the FDA as a sleeping medication, but the bad news is that it requires a prescription—a bit more expensive and inconvenient, but prompting more trust in the ingredients. Ramelteon has been shown to be effective in insomnia and in circadian rhythm disorders as well.

The public uses melatonin mostly as a sleep-inducing agent, not so much as a circadian rhythm-changing agent, which takes more information for proper use than most people have access to. Based on dozens of letters in response to newspaper articles on melatonin, it appears that some people are very satisfied with melatonin, feeling that it puts them to sleep quickly; others feel that it doesn't help much; and some complain of side effects, particularly vivid nightmares.

What are the reasons for these discrepancies?

For one, there seems to be no public standard for dose or time of dosage, so these could affect response; one must also consider *what else* might be in their particular over-the-counter "melatonin" that could play a role in efficacy or side effects. Getting a "verified" product may help in avoiding these problems.

As for dosage and time of dosing: I would suggest 3–5 mg to achieve the sleepiness effect, and always aim for the lowest effective dose, and taking it 15 minutes before bedtime would seem logical for use as an hypnotic. Other instructions (such as three hours before bedtime) may be appropriate for use in people with delayed sleep phase syndrome, which is another problem entirely.

There is now a new role for melatonin, one that is potentially life-saving, and that is as a "cytoprotective" drug in the treatment of REM sleep behavior disorder (RBD). "Cytoprotective" means protecting cells, in this case brain cells that deteriorate in RBD, generally over a decade or so, resulting in dementia and eventually in death. Very high doses (60–100mg) may be necessary for this treatment. We will discuss this in more detail in the section on RBD.

Orexin antagonists: You may recall from the section on narcolepsy (see page 156) that orexin is a natural neurotransmitter thought to produce alertness. A profound deficiency of orexin causes type I narcolepsy, a disorder involving serious daytime sleepiness. Once orexin was understood to prevent sleepiness, it made sense to wonder if *blocking* its effects in the brain could produce sleepiness when sleepiness was most desired, as in insomnia patients. And so the hypnotics in the category of orexin-blockers were born (well, developed).

These new drugs—called *dual orexin receptor antagonists* (DORAs), as they block both forms of orexin—go by the chemical (brand) names like suvorexant (Belsomra) and lemorexant (Dayvigo). They have proved to be effective for some patients with insomnia (approved, as always, for short term use). Insurance coverage for newer drugs can always be problematic, however, so these can be expensive if coverage is denied.

DORAs may prove to be safer than the benzos over the next few years, but we must reserve judgment for this given the experience with benzos—remember, it took decades to understand the dangers of benzos. There is one set of side effects that is specific to this group that is worth knowing: narcolepsy-like symptoms. Narcolepsy is characterized by abnormally low orexin levels; in fact, the lower the level, the more severe is the narcolepsy and the sleepiness that accompanies it. Orexin antagonists block the orexin receptors in the brain, essentially telling the receptors that the orexin levels are low even when they aren't.

Orexin blockers produce sleepiness by mimicking narcolepsy, so it's not surprising that they can produce some of the complications of narcolepsy in normal patients: cataplexy (sudden localized muscle weakness), hallucinations, and sleep paralysis (see page 159). These occur in a small percentage of people who take orexin antagonists, but they and their physicians may be perplexed when these unusual side effects occur, so "forewarned is forearmed." A good discussion of possible side effects may prevent future anxiety.

There is one other side effect of sleeping pills (hypnotics) that is worth mentioning: "complex sleep behaviors." This can be thought of as "drug-induced sleepwalking." We will discuss sleepwalking in detail later in this book (Chapter Six), but all forms of abnormal behavior during sleep that we call "sleepwalking" can occur in people who have no history of sleepwalking but then do bizarre activities during sleep after taking one of these drugs.

This problem is relatively rare but potentially serious: it includes sleep-related walking, eating, and driving, with associated risks of injuries, falls, drowning, car accidents, burns, and death. It has been reported after the use of benzo-receptor agonists (Ambien, Lunesta, and Sonata) and with the orexin-blockers (Belsomra and Dayvigo), but appears less likely with the standard benzos, antihistamines, antipsychotics, antidepressants, and melatonin.

I have painted a pretty grim picture of sleeping pills. Admittedly, I am not a fan! But I must admit that a small minority of patients I have seen with insomnia have claimed to do well after many years of taking a particular drug. My innate skepticism leads me to ask what would happen to these few if they tried to stop the medication, but that isn't something they were interested in—they felt that they were doing just fine, and were happy with taking their sleeping pill nightly for the rest of their lives. I had to wonder, however, how long they could continue to do that without tolerance or withdrawal symptoms.

Even in the absence of those, the risk of incipient dementia hovers over the whole idea. Were they at increased risk for dementia? If their preferred drug was a benzodiazepine, the answer might be: yes. Did they have a family history of dementia? (It's depressingly common.) Occasionally fear of this terrible outcome is enough to persuade someone to work their way off these hypnotics, but not always.

There is recent information[78] suggesting that DORAs may be useful in weaning addicted patients off benzos, especially when combined with

CBTi (see below). The appearance of articles like this brightens my day because it illustrates that there is increasing awareness in the medical community and in the public at large of the dangers of prolonged hypnotic use, of the potential for avoidance of some of those problems, and of the prime value of CBTi.

Let's talk about CBTi now.

A panacea for our time

As mentioned earlier, *CBTi* is cognitive behavioral therapy for insomnia. There is help in the mental health community using regular CBT (without the "i") for many psychologic problems: anxiety from various causes, such as fear of flying or fear of needles, as well as for anxiety of unknown cause; depression, post-traumatic stress disorder, attention-deficit disorder, eating disorders, and so forth. Many psychologists and counselors are trained in CBT for a whole range of problems, but it turns out that CBT for insomnia—*CBTi*—requires special training in understanding the psychology of sleep—so searching out a specialist in this category is usually necessary.

CBTi in general is a "talk-therapy" process, called goal-oriented because it is not a Woody Allen-like 20-year form of psychotherapy that potentially could last a lifetime. Instead, it is usually a structured program lasting a few weeks or so, aimed at fixing a particular problem. It involves reviewing negative thought patterns and unhelpful behavioral responses to the problem; frequently an examination of self-image, social and family relationships, and even our worldview come into play.

With regard to the specific program of CBT for insomnia, it seeks to explore the negative thought patterns that produce or perpetuate insomnia, as well as unhelpful responses to insomnia that may make sleeping less likely rather than more. Of course, underlying anxieties, depression, and other mental issues must be taken into account if they play a role here, and occasionally "escalation" of therapy to a psychiatrist is helpful. But for the most part, CBTi has dramatically changed our approach to insomnia over the last 20 years.

For the last few years, CBTi has been considered "first-line therapy" for chronic insomnia. This means that CBTi is the first approach to be considered for most people with chronic insomnia, *not* hypnotic medications, particularly not open-ended (long-term) hypnotics. This shift is in recognition of the limitations and complications of hypnotics as primary treatment for insomnia.

It's hard to overemphasize the significance of the sea change that this new approach represents: for the first time in over 50 years, medications are *not* considered the best way to treat this problem. The standard practice for thousands of doctors treating millions of patients is now changing, and for the better. Research has shown that CBTi has better short-term, and more importantly, better long-term results with insomnia, and with fewer complications and side effects.

Let's look at the basic elements of CBTi, and perhaps we can understand why it is so helpful.

Sleep hygiene is a strange term, seeming to refer to the "cleanliness" of sleep, but it really means good habits of sleep, habits that promote falling asleep easily and maintaining sleep in good quantity and quality so that one feels refreshed and alert after sleep, so that the healthful effects that sleep has to offer can be achieved. Sleep logs and sleep diaries may be useful in establishing a baseline for these habits.

We know from our earlier discussions of normal sleep and the consequences of insufficient sleep how important the choices we make—about the timing of our sleep, about our sleep environment, and about our behaviors before sleep—can affect the amount and quality of the sleep we achieve, and the consequences of those choices in how we feel during the day. Here are some of the mainstays of sleep hygiene that are likely to be discussed with every patient undergoing CBTi:

1. Try to maintain the same bedtime and the same risetime daily.

2. Recognize the effects of caffeine on your particular system, and limit use no later than that which might inhibit sleep.

3. Understand that alcohol promotes awakenings and poor sleep in the second half of the night, and limit alcohol use appropriately in the hours before sleep.

4. Limit food intake in the hours before sleep.

5. Avoid bright light late in the evenings, whether from lighting sources or from screens.

6. Try to increase bright light exposure in the mornings and enforce darkness during sleep.

7. Plan tasks requiring focused attention in the mornings and aim for quiet distraction in the hours before retiring.

These rules seem basic and simple, and they might be considered easy to follow until one adds in social, family, work, and medical constraints. How hard is it to maintain the same bedtime when one works rotating shifts? How does one limit alcohol when it is part of an active social life, or just a habit? How does one get bright light in the mornings when one drives to work early, in the dark? How does one relax before bedtime with four teenage boys in the house? And so forth.

How the messiness of our day-to-day lives complicates these guidelines is a challenge for sleep psychologists daily. When these goals are aspired to and sometimes actually achieved, patients improve.

Sleep restriction means limiting time in bed closer to the time of actual sleep. We read an example of this in the story of 24-year-old Frank (see page 198) who responded to difficulty sleeping, as people frequently do, by increasing his hours in bed, which paradoxically made his insomnia worse. His approach served to give him more hours in bed awake, more hours obsessing about how to get to sleep, but no more minutes of actual sleep.

The opposite approach is to limit the hours in bed to something close to the number of hours of actual sleep; this means more time out of bed in the evening, awake, which promotes more sleep during the shorter hours in bed by increasing "sleep pressure" on the brain. Once those hours in bed are almost full of sleep, the time in bed can be extended and a deeper night of sleep achieved.

In some cases of insomnia, sleep restriction is the only technique necessary to revert to normal sleep. When this approach works, its success is frequently a pleasant surprise to the sleeper. Combined with other aspects of sleep hygiene, it's even more effective.

Stimulus control is based on the theory that using the bed as a venue for more things than just sleep and sex (for example, as a place for laptop work, watching TV, reading, playing board games, eating meals, making business calls, and so forth) can confuse our minds when we try to relax, let go, and fall asleep in that same bed. If we retrain our brains to think of the bed as *the place for sleep* and nothing else, the stimulus of getting in bed will more likely elicit the response of feeling sleepy and then falling asleep.

The first step is to avoid all uses of the bed for non-sleep/non-sex activities, and for those who find themselves unable to fall sleep for more than 15–20 minutes at the beginning of the night, or tossing and turning in bed for hours, the idea is to leave the bed and the bedroom, to go to another room and do some calming activity, like reading something not too exciting, in dim light. (The rationale for dim light is prevent the alerting effect of bright light.) Once sleepiness begins, returning to the bed is allowed, and hopefully sleep is then achieved. The same approach is used for prolonged middle-of-the-night awakenings. Multiple out-of-bed episodes may be needed on some nights.

This can be a tough guideline to follow. It's not fun to leave a nice warm bed and go to another room, insomnia notwithstanding. It may be boring to read something unstimulating (that is, something boring) in dim light, while wishing one was back in bed. But this guideline remains in the recommendations because it works. It's part of the long game in fighting insomnia, in that it takes some time, a number of nights of practicing this, to achieve *control* of the stimulus, to the point where being in bed becomes the stimulus for sleep rather than for the anxiety for sleep. Once successful, it can lead to improved sleep with little need to leave the bedroom over time.

Cognitive restructuring involves exploration of thought patterns that emerge around sleep struggles, understanding negative and counterproductive ideas that worsen insomnia ("I'll never get to sleep." "I'll be a wreck all day tomorrow if I don't go to sleep right now." "I know sleep loss causes depression and anxiety and dementia. Am I getting those?" "I've been lying here for hours trying to sleep and only 20 minutes have passed on my bedside clock.").

Once these thoughts are identified, they can be supplanted by positive responses ("It may take me a while to fall asleep, but I'll still be OK tomorrow." "Everybody has problems sleeping sometime; this is not that abnormal." "Even after a bad night I know I've still gotten some hours of sleep, so I'll just do better next time." "I know it's likely I'll think in the morning that I haven't slept at all, when in reality I will have acquired a few hours of sleep at least.") Guided discovery is used to help the patient challenge dysfunctional thoughts and understand more realistic and less-threatening concepts of sleep.

Relaxation training includes many techniques of "letting go." Some people respond best to relaxation at bedtime, others earlier in the evenings, and some use it in the middle of the night after arousals. There are dozens of ways to promote relaxation, from progressive muscle relaxation (flexing and relaxing muscles from the feet to the head), breathing patterns (deep breathing, diaphragmatic breathing, guided breathing), mindfulness and meditation. There are dozens of passive and guided meditation apps on the internet now. Other options include podcasts with narratives, speech, and music on the internet, anything that achieves distraction and allows the brain to disconnect.

How does one pursue cognitive behavioral therapy for insomnia? I liken this quest to a simpler situation: suppose you were charged with having to pass a physics exam in six weeks, but you had never taken physics before, and this is not enough time for an ordinary course in physics. Your choices are: buy the physics textbook on which the test is based; take an internet-based course, maybe one taught by the actual author of that textbook; or meet daily one-on-one with a physics teacher, in person, addressing all aspects of physics that might be on the test. If you guessed that the last choice is the best, I agree.

With insomnia, you could approach treatment by buying the textbook (in this case, one of the best is *Say Goodnight to Insomnia,* by Gregg Jacobs), taking an internet-based CBTi course (such as on Dr Jacobs' website, at *cbtforinsomnia.com,* or other programs like "Sleepio," "Stellar Sleep," "Insomnia Coach," and others), or seeking out a specially trained, CBTi-certified sleep psychologist who will meet with you individually, in person or virtually, to pursue CBTi over a period of weeks.

In my experience over the past 30 years as a sleep physician, certified sleep psychologists are worth their weight in gold. Success rates with insomnia, particularly chronic insomnia, increased dramatically in the early 2000s when CBTi became available, and medication-based treatments started to fade in popularity. Now, 20+ years into this approach, sleep physicians and many primary care physicians turn to CBTi first for treatment of difficult insomnia.

The biggest hurdle was, and remains, the lack of large numbers of certified sleep psychologists, a problem that is somewhat ameliorated by the availability of virtual sessions, making geography less of a challenge, and internet-based programs. And while you might learn more physics one-on-one with a tutor in person than online, internet-based CBTi has been shown to produce almost as good results as in-person treatment, even, in some cases, when anxiety or depression play a role.[79] It's certainly worth considering.

So what would I recommend for insomnia now? It depends entirely on severity, which in the case of insomnia means it depends on the degree of desperation. The most severe insomnia engenders the most desperate need for help, for "just a little sleep." This group is best served by in-person treatment (virtual or actual), because they really need *someone to talk to*, someone who'll listen. It's arguable that these unfortunate patients have the most anxiety, which is not uncommonly a chicken–egg issue about which came first, though at some point it no longer matters. They need to talk, they need help, and they need to sleep. A sleep physician can recommend an hypnotic while they are arranging their CBTi, though typically they have already tried most hypnotics on the market by the time they are seen. So for this desperate group, I strongly recommend in-person CBTi if possible; if not, go directly to the internet.

For moderate insomnia, for the unhappy-but-not-really-desperate sleeper, the internet approach is a good place to start. Some of these involve feedback from human sleep professionals, approximating the individual attention available from in-person therapy.

For mild insomnia, of recent onset even if occasionally recurrent, one might start with Dr Jacob's book alone. The basic concepts of CBTi are there, described by one of the originators of the process; many of my patients found this immensely helpful. If more help is needed, an internet-based program is likely to help.

Overall CBTi has a reported success rate of 70–80%. In previous decades, nothing like that was ever achieved with hypnotic medication therapy (particularly not in the long term), so we are delighted that this technique is available to us. Medications still play a role, especially in the short-term treatment of insomnia, but long-term?

We now have a better approach.

What about that last 20% who do not respond to CBTi? Many of these have "comorbid" issues that may complicate cognitive therapy by inhibiting relaxation techniques or interfering with cognitive restructuring—problems like ADHD, PTSD, severe anxiety or depression, bipolar disease, psychosis, or alcohol or drug dependency. It's important that other sleep problems are not ignored (particularly obstructive sleep apnea and restless legs syndrome) in this group, and that ongoing attention is given to their mental issues as well as sleep complaints.

Insomnia can be transient and mild, or chronic and in some cases life-disrupting. Cognitive behavioral therapy is by far the best option in the more difficult situations. Exclusion of other sleep disorders is also key. A sleep physician and a qualified sleep psychologist make the best team in these situations. The classic approach with long-term sleeping pills should be avoided if possible.

But I don't feel old...

Some people sleep better than others, and this is true with sleep as we age. The way human sleep patterns change as we get older will affect all of us…if we're lucky enough to get to that age we call "elderly." Some consider anyone older than 55 to be in that category; some use 65 as a cutoff. But as we are generally so much healthier now in most ways after middle age (whatever *that* is) than previous generations were, we tend to think of "elderly" as later and later, older and older, maybe only when one is more feeble and frail.

Those in age groups previously qualifying as elderly now seem more vigorous and healthy, thanks to better diets, more exercise, better sleep habits (!), better air quality, less smoking, more health-consciousness, and to some degree to more plastic surgery. But this goes only so far. As one wit recently observed, "Fifty is the new 40, and 60 is the new 50, but 70 isn't the new anything." Age does catch up with us all at some point, and it's quite clear that we all age at different rates, depending on our genetics, our environment, a lifetime of our behaviors, and just plain luck.

Here are two histograms (maps of sleep stages, or sleep architecture) comparing the sleep of a typical person in their 40s and one in their 70s (we're ignoring gender):

The first thing to notice is that the sleep period length is longer in the younger person: the younger person in this example is sleeping from

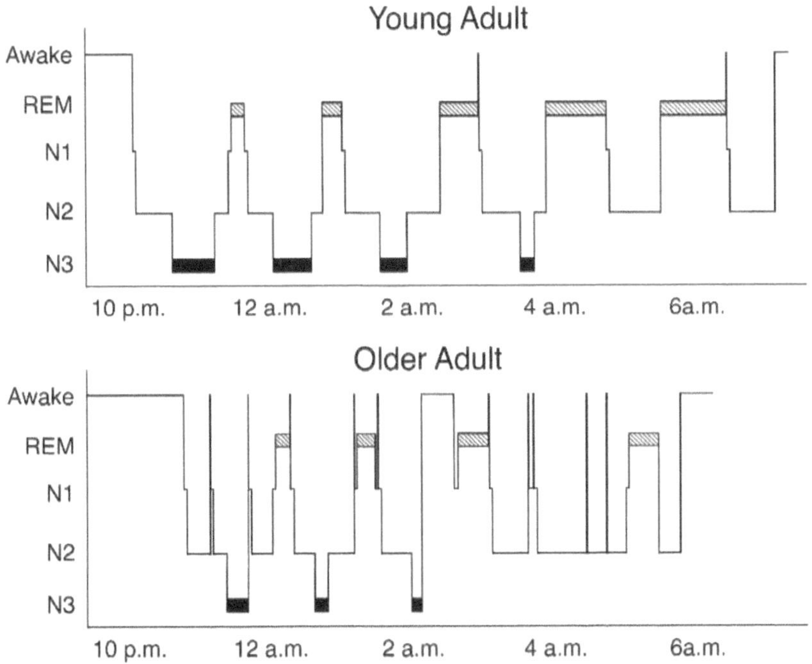

FIGURE 5. Sleep histograms for young and older adults. See text below for discussion.

10pm to 7am; the older person is sleeping less overall. We know that older people have a form of advanced sleep phase syndrome, meaning that they have a tendency to go to bed earlier and awaken earlier than they did when they were younger. This change appears to be a function of an aging circadian regulatory system in the brain, as well as a drop in the overall amount of melatonin that is produced nightly.

The result is a sleep phase (the timing of sleep in the light-dark cycle) that is *advanced*, or earlier, both in its onset (when sleep starts) and off-set (when final wake occurs). With an advanced phase, one feels the need to go to bed earlier and to wake earlier than previously. All other things being equal, the overall amount of sleep should not change, but just occur sooner.

But it does change, and in lots of ways. Some elders have more difficulty going to sleep; most have lots of awakenings—very brief and/or much longer ones—during the night; some have difficulty with even earlier morning awakenings; and some have all these problems. We can see these in the histogram of the elderly above: the amount of time to fall asleep (sleep latency) is longer than in the younger person's histogram; there are more very brief awakenings and some longer ones; and the time of final awakening is earlier.

There are lots of reasons why these things happen to us as we age, and these fall into specific categories.

Habits we've acquired—or lost. Why do the elderly have difficulty falling asleep and more awakenings? The simple answer appears to be that they are *stimulated* more—by pain (such as arthritis or reflux), by discomfort (such as the need to urinate), by chemicals (alcohol, nicotine), and perhaps by the anxieties and regrets of life. We have the sense that our sleep becomes more fragile, more easily disturbed as we age, so adding anything to that tendency that promotes arousals will make sleep quality worse.

Notice on the two histograms above the difference in the amount of deep (N3): on the elderly person's histogram, there is none. Remember from our previous discussions how important deep sleep is (see pages 69 and 77) in terms of sleep quality and restorative sleep, particularly in the "cleansing of the brain" that deep sleep and removal of beta-amyloid from the brain.* And recall that the things that most promote deep sleep are adolescence (teens get large amounts of N3 sleep), sleep deprivation, and exercise.

---

* See page 74. Although we have recently learned that beta-amyloid (which is associated with the brain pathology of the dementia of Alzheimer's disease) is cleared from the brain much more during deep sleep, we are still a few giant steps from proving that getting more deep sleep can prevent—or improve, or even stabilize—dementia. My guess is that it can, and it generally won't hurt to try, but recent research on Alzheimer's patients with drugs that purport to reduce beta-amyloid in the brain have been disappointing, failing to show improvements in cognitive function. Much more needs to be done to understand these relationships.

For our elderly, the only logical way to get more deep sleep is to get more exercise (whether resistance, aerobic, or a mixture of the two). We noted earlier that deep sleep "normally" seems to begin to diminish on sleep studies in patients as young as their 40's—could this be related to a tendency after that age to exercise less? Certainly that would be likely in the 70–80-year-old group. They may no longer be exercising at the level they might have been half a century earlier.

Many of them can't exercise much at all, given other health issues like arthritis, old injuries, surgeries, and so forth, but for the rest, an introduction into exercise with gradual increases in timing and intensity may be a valid way to promote N3 sleep. This can help with the overall quality of sleep. On the internet now there are lots of exercise programs for the elderly and the previously sedentary that are easily downloadable and are simple to perform. Paradoxically, the greatest risk of any exercise program is injury, which can prevent further exercise and promote more of a sedentary existence, so the word *gradual* cannot be emphasized enough in planning such a program.

Smoking and alcohol use both adversely affect sleep, and both result in early morning awakenings, potentially worsening that tendency of the elderly to wake more frequently in the second half of the night. As is true in younger people, alcohol causes earlier awakenings by being metabolized into "alerting substances;" it's common for all of us to fall asleep more quickly after drinking alcohol, but then to wake at 4–5am, perhaps fully alert and unable to return to sleep, the next day. Nicotine causes awakenings at all ages through nicotine withdrawal: while daytime withdrawal symptoms can be assuaged by smoking every few minutes or hours, nighttime symptoms may become more intense unless one awakes every few hours to smoke, to replenish that falling nicotine level. Nicotine withdrawal diminishes both sleep quality and quantity, which may even result in daytime sleepiness.

Other sleep disorders. One very common sleep disorder that must be considered with almost any sleep complaint in the elderly is obstructive sleep apnea (see page 129); another somewhat less common one is restless legs syndrome, or RLS (see page 184). As with many medical diagnoses, these problems can sometimes be subtle and may not be easily apparent to the patient (elderly or not) nor to their families. RLS is diagnosed by history (that is, asking the right questions—there is no test for this) while sleep apnea, sometimes suspected by history, requires some form of sleep study for confirmation.

Both of these illnesses can cause difficulty falling asleep and more awakenings later in the night. Both can cause unrefreshing sleep and daytime sleepiness. Treatment of either is usually straightforward and can produce dramatic improvements in sleep and the priceless sense of daytime wellbeing.

Bad luck illnesses. Anyone fighting a significant disease or injury over time may develop difficulty sleeping as a result, whether from anxiety and/or depression over the severity and worrisome threats of the illness, from the pain or discomfort arising from the illness itself, or from the side effects of the treatments of these illnesses.

These problems are obviously not limited to the elderly—but some older people say they are just waiting for that next shoe to fall, that next illness to appear, that next medication they must take and that next side effect they must weather. This is perhaps one of the origins of the expression, "Getting old is not for sissies." At the same time, when questioned as to whether they wish to continue living, the answer is almost always "Yes!" Giving up is rarely the option chosen.

Many elderly describe a sense of acceptance of their limitations and disabilities, and also describe a level of happiness one might not predict, given these problems. A certain wisdom arises from years of experience and understanding the ways of human nature and life itself. How we as individuals deal with the slings and arrows of life's fortunes determines not only how well we sleep at night, but how satisfied we are with our lot throughout the day as well.

The aches and pains of getting old. The well-known "aches and pains" of the elderly are not the same in everyone. Some of this discomfort is attributed to loss of flexibility over time of tendons and ligaments, causing stiffness and pain; some is attributed to the triad of "osteopenia, osteoporosis, and osteoarthritis." Osteopenia means loss of bone structure, mild in degree; osteoporosis is the same thing, but more moderate to severe (in severe cases, it can lead to fractures).

Osteoarthritis is pain within the joints, traditionally described as "wear and tear arthritis," which can sound dismissive ("Why can't you just accept that it's part of getting old?"). There are treatments for loss of bone (exercise, vitamin D, sunlight, calcium, medications), just as there are for osteoarthritis (exercise, anti-inflammatories, weight loss, even joint replacement surgeries), so hope is not lost. In the meantime, however, pain during sleep can be disruptive, leading to multiple arousals and insufficient sleep.

Anxiety and depression. Anxiety at any age may result in insomnia—sleep-onset or sleep-maintenance or both—and that type of insomnia may be harder to treat until the underlying anxiety is addressed. The same is true of depression in the elderly, but this is a bit harder to assess sometimes as an older person with depression may not look like a younger one would: they may be more withdrawn or uninterested in being active, rather than appearing sad or depressed. An open mind in diagnosing, and a low bar for testing for depression in the elderly can be revealing.

Recommendations. What, therefore, might I suggest for the elderly in general to pursue better sleep?

Similar things, perhaps, to those suggested for everyone else with difficulty sleeping (as in the previous section on insomnia), and a few things that apply specifically to the aged:

1. **Exercise**

   This is such an important recommendation, knowing as we do that deep sleep is prompted by exercise, that overall sleep quality and quantity can improve with exercise. Even small amounts of aerobic or resistance exercise have positive results in cardiovascular fitness, sense of well-being, joint and muscle strength, and longevity. For those with significant disabilities, unable perhaps to run or even walk, there may yet be benefits from isometric or isotonic exercises.

Again, a gently increasing level of exercise is important to prevent injury. Starting with a short walk around the house is a good first step for some. A visit to a good physical therapist for customized recommendations can be very helpful. A good program of stretching, such as yoga, may help with the problem of stiffness in aging tissues. All of this can result in improved sleep, improved mood and sense of well-being during the day.

2. **Sunlight**

Morning sunlight is frequently recommended for those with insomnia, as it not only acts to reset the circadian pacemaker each morning but also improves mood and alertness. In the elderly, however, when an advanced sleep phase (feeling a strong impulse to go to bed in the evenings and get up in the mornings much earlier than desired) is an issue, sunlight in the late afternoon and evening, if available, is even better than morning sunlight. In this setting, seasonal evening sunlight helps delay the sleep phase, pushing bedtimes and risetime to later points, making bedtimes and risetimes more normal and in keeping with those of the rest of society.

The brightness of sunlight so exceeds that of most indoor lighting that its shifting effect is greater than most any set of lightbulbs, and sunlight's ability to improve mood and alertness remains. Wearing "blue-blocker" sunglasses is *not* recommended, by the way, as this screens out the spectrum of sunlight that most improves sleep timing. Of course, one should *never* look directly into the sun, but should sunshine be considered harmful otherwise? Yes—the UV radiation is what causes skin cancer and skin aging, as well as cataracts (see page 90). If you haven't had cataract surgery, UV-blocking sunglasses may be a good preventative of cataracts, even if those glasses diminish your ability to use sunlight to its maximum benefit for circadian rhythm maintenance.

3. **Medications**

   Consider the possibility that your medications can affect sleep. Ask your doctor if any of your medicines have side effects such as insomnia or awakenings. A trial time off a questionable medicine may clarify this. Any medicines or supplements that contain caffeine (as in migraine medicines) or vasoconstrictors, like ephedrine (as in some allergy medicines) can inhibit sleep.

   As for aches and pains during the night, an anti-inflammatory medication (for example, ibuprofen) or analgesic (like Tylenol) at bedtime can make a big difference in sleep quality if pain is an issue (or if you just suspect it—pain can cause arousals of which you may not be aware). The caveat here—and this must be said strongly—is that most anti-inflammatories can cause kidney problems, particularly in those over 65, so a nightly dose should not be started without the approval of one's physician. Medications specifically for osteoporosis, such as bisphosphonates, may help over time with pain, by slowing or reversing bone loss. Vitamin D is an important medication for this, too, as it helps with calcium metabolism in bones.

4. **Other sleep disorders**

   Be sure there are no underlying sleep disorders, such as sleep apnea (do you snore? Stop breathing during the night? Feel sleepy much of the day?) or RLS (do weird sensations in your legs keep you awake or wake you up at night?). If there is any question of one of these, seek out a sleep physician's help.

5. **Other illnesses**

   Other illnesses that result in pain or side effects of medications can frequently be improved by medication adjustments or other treatments, but not unless they are addressed. Don't hesitate to tell your physician that sleep seems to be affected by your illness or medications; with the emphasis on the importance of sleep as a part of good health considerations now, most physicians will find resources to help you if you alert them to this issue.

6. **Anxiety and depression**

Keep an open mind about these possibilities. Seek help if there is any question of anxiety or depression; therapy can change your sleep and can change your life. Remember that sleep and anxiety/depression are bidirectional, meaning that difficulty with sleep can worsen anxiety and depression, and anxiety and depression can make sleep problems worse. Sometimes both must be addressed simultaneously—which is a good thing, since they may be two different problems. Be assertive about this, as the payoff can be large. Don't assume that someone else will make you do it.

PEARLS OF WISDOM

All of us will experience changes in our sleep patterns in older age, just as we all do in puberty. These changes can be managed with good behavioral practices (avoiding smoking, and alcohol, getting appropriate exercise and sunlight exposure, keeping good sleep habits) and watching for medication side effects.

CHAPTER 6

Things that Go Bump in the Night

Sleepwalking

Sleepwalking is the closest we humans come to being zombies.* The traditional zombie of myth, centuries ago, was a person who had died and then was revived from the dead by magic, most commonly black magic or voodoo in Africa or Haiti. The zombie is "undead," acting partially alive (able to move, though not very well; able to verbalize, though not very well; seemingly on some sort of quest, like murder) and partially dead (not very responsive to their environment, not likely ever to come back to "normal").

 Sleepwalking competes with dreaming as the most "storied" of all aspects of sleep. We have all heard stories of famous people who were sleepwalkers, like Nancy Reagan, Jennifer Aniston, and the comedian Mike Birbiglia.[80] There seems to be no limit as to the behaviors people have been reported to do while sleeping: walking, running, eating, searching, urinating, jumping out of windows, driving, even engaging in sexual or in some cases violent acts.

---

* There is at least one major difference: most zombies, particularly on TV and in movies, stagger when they walk. Sleepwalkers, on the other hand, seem to exhibit a good sense of balance.

All of these behaviors come under the category of *complex behaviors,* with movements we could think of as having some basic purpose. Contrast these to *simple behaviors,* which do not seem to have much purpose, like talking and rolling over in bed. *Sleep-talking,* which is very common, is now considered a normal variant of sleep, not a disorder. If your bedpartner does this, enjoy it. It's not an illness.

Sleepwalking is a form of **parasomnia**, which means *abnormal behavior during sleep.* We divide parasomnias into those that "jump out" of REM sleep and those that "jump out" of non-REM sleep. Let's start with the parasomnias that happen out of non-REM sleep, the most common of which is sleepwalking.

Non-REM parasomnias

Abnormal behaviors arising from non-REM sleep occur coming out of deep (N3) sleep, not transitional (N1) sleep or light (N2) sleep. You may recall from Chapter One that deep sleep normally involves movement of the body in bed (in the case of children, lots of movement) and, compared to REM sleep, involves less brain blood flow, lower brain temperature, and lower brain electrical activity. (I mentioned in Chapter One that we loosely refer to N3 sleep as "active body, dead brain.") So these abnormal behaviors are starting out of a state where the brain is inactive, and doesn't like to wake up quickly. People awakened from deep sleep say, "It was so hard to wake up. I just couldn't jumpstart my brain fast enough."

Gloria, a 27-year-old secretary, began having episodes every few months during her teens described by family and later by her husband Chris as suddenly sitting up in bed, moving her arms about randomly, sometimes moving her legs, moaning a bit, and then going back to sleep. The episodes lasted no more than one to two minutes, and she never remembered them the next morning, or even a few minutes later if Chris awakened her. He noticed that the episodes occurred mostly in the first few hours of sleep.

Dr. Smith, a sleep physician, reassured the couple that she had confusional arousals, that they were harmless and not likely to lead to overt sleepwalking, and that they would likely tail off in frequency as she approached her 40s. This turned out to be exactly what happened.

We think of two categories of these non-REM parasomnias: those where the sleeper stays in bed, and those where they leave the bed. If the sleeper stays in bed with their unusual behavior, it's called a *confusional arousal,* a variant of which is *sleep-sex*; if they leave the bed, it's either *sleepwalking* or one of its variants: *sleep-eating* or *sleep terrors.*

The onset of any of these tends to be sudden, an abrupt jump from deep sleep into something else, something lighter. One moment the sleeper is peacefully asleep in deep sleep, and the next moment they are "aroused," meaning that they are moving about but not entirely awake, not interacting normally with their environment, but seemingly moving toward awakening. They may suddenly sit up in bed, open their eyes with a "glassy stare," move their arms around, say a few nonsensical words and seem confused, shift their body somewhat, then lie down after a minute or so and go back to sleep.

But they *stay in bed.*

We call this brief episode a **confusional arousal**, not rising to the level of "sleepwalking" mainly because the sleeper never left the bed. Both confusional arousals and sleepwalking are similar, both arising out of deep sleep and ending in wake or lighter non-REM sleep (N1 or N2), and both followed by, for the sleeper, little or no memory of the event.

Confusional arousals are said to be normal in children under the age of three, and less so later. As my two children were growing up, I'm sure they had episodes of confusional arousals, though Monica and I would not have known it unless we happened to be right at the bedside when one occurred. Most would have occurred out of our presence, but we might not have thought much of one even had we been there to see the whole event, as the activity might not seem that unusual.

Perhaps 4% of all adults have confusional arousals. Having an underlying issue with anxiety or depression increases the odds that these might happen. These episodes are generally harmless and require no intervention at all.

Indulge me in a walk down Memory Lane. In the 1980s I loved driving my Datsun 240Z, the last manual transmission car I ever owned. Over a few years' time it started making more noises when I shifted into third gear, but after a little grinding, it seemed to move into shift fully and to drive well. Then one day a friend pointed out to me that it needed to be repaired. The problem had come on so gradually that I had missed it.

After third gear was replaced, I was delighted to find that it shifted so much better, and humbled that it took me so long to realize the problem was in the transmission. One expects one's car's transmission to make smooth shifts from, say, first into second and second to third, but in my unrepaired 240Z, I frequently got stuck between second and third as the gears grinded loudly. I was caught in a border zone between the two gears, and could not drive. After replacing the gears, I could confidently drive in second or third and not get stuck in between.

The brain has a similar transmission function when it comes to sleep. It wants to make quick and complete shifts from one sleep stage to the next. Look back at a sleep histogram (see page 33) and think of the brain's role in shifting from wake to stage N1 (transitional sleep) to stage N2 (light sleep), then to stage N3 (deep sleep), and later into REM. It's shifting constantly throughout the night.

Parasomnias are thought to represent an immaturity or fragility of the brain's ability to shift between sleep stages, specifically between deep sleep and wake. Remember, this is hard for everyone. But in those with those with non-REM parasomnias, the shift sometimes is incomplete, and they're caught in the middle. They're not fully awake nor fully asleep. Research has shown EEG evidence of continued sleep in some parts of the brain, and of wake in other parts (especially the motor parts) in sleepwalkers, which fits our concept of an incomplete shift.

All of us are subject to triggers that might cause arousals during sleep. It might be a sound in the bedroom or from outside, an internal sensation (like a full bladder), or something more subtle, maybe something internal that we don't know how to detect. In normal sleepers, that something might cause an arousal or an awakening (arousals are shorter), meaning a shift from deep sleep to wake, or just a shift to a lighter stage, say N1 or N2, and nothing else, and then…back to sleep.

But consider a child with a family history of sleepwalking who has herself shown confusional arousals in the past. If she is exposed to a sound or other stimulus while in deep sleep, for example, normally she might shift to a lighter stage briefly and then return to deep sleep when no longer stimulated, and never show much movement.

But at other times things go awry. Her brain's attempt to shift from deep sleep to a lighter stage malfunctions and is incomplete; her brain shows aspects of wake, like open eyes, vague talking, and semi-purposeful muscle movements, but some aspects of sleep too, like seeming confused during the event, being poorly responsive to questions, and showing no memory of the whole event afterwards. (In small children, loud, inconsolable screaming is also common.) Within a few minutes, she shifts back to a normal non-REM stage, and is peacefully asleep again.

This theory is that her sleep-stage shifting system is not fully formed, not yet mature. This theory is attractive but probably overly simplistic. But as a concept it helps us understand why confusional arousals become less frequent in older children and especially in adults, as their brains mature and the borders between their sleep stages become better defined, so they can respond to arousals during sleep with more appropriate shifts to other stages—and back.

The same concept applies to **sleepwalking**, that category of abnormal sleep behaviors involving leaving the bed. Sleepwalking runs in families, and frequently starts in childhood, so by adulthood we usually know who the sleepwalkers are. Sleepwalking is less common after age eight, but may persist into adolescence and beyond. Maybe 4% of all adults sleepwalk, but many are not reported.

Lonnie was told by his family that he began sleepwalking around age 11. His parents were not surprised by this as his father had been a sleepwalker until his 40s. On occasion his parents awakened to find him in their bedroom in the middle of the night, walking around with a blank stare, reacting minimally to their questions. At times he appeared to be searching for something behind a chair or bed. They learned to gently guide him back to his bed, where he rapidly went back to sleep; he was always surprised the next day when they described what happened the night before, as he could not remember any of it.

His sleepwalking episodes became less frequent over time, and were never a problem for him.

Remember that the sleepwalker themselves will not remember the activity unless they are fully awakened from it away from the bed; sleepwalking in one or more family members may be harmless and even considered entertaining in the family lore, and may not require medical attention unless harms occur. Since the normal amounts of deep sleep diminish as we age, sleepwalking frequency seems to lessen after age 40. This can be encouraging to a person approaching middle age who hopes his or her sleepwalking will stop at some point.

As non-REM parasomnias, sleepwalking and confusional arousals occur out of deep sleep and therefore usually occur in the first third of the night, as that is when most deep sleep takes place (children and younger adults can have deep sleep later in the night too). In evaluating abnormal sleep behaviors, sleep doctors always want to know at what point in the sleep cycle the problem occurs. REM-related parasomnias are most likely in the last third of the night, as this is when most normal REM occurs. Sleepwalking episodes last as little as a minute but can run 10 minutes or longer.

Roger was 35 when his wife Ellen began noticing his sleepwalking. A few times a month, after one to two hours of sleep, he would get out of bed and walk around his bedroom, occasionally going downstairs to the kitchen or living room. He never disturbed anything in the house and seemed to handle stairs well. Ellen took him to Dr. Smith, the sleep physician, who made note of Roger's recent weight gain and heard from Ellen that Roger had begun snoring and snorting during sleep over the past year.

Dr. Smith obtained a sleep study that showed mild obstructive sleep apnea, with breathing interruptions an average of 14 times an hour. Roger was reluctant to consider CPAP for this sleep apnea (after all, he had gone to the doctor to discuss sleepwalking!), but once accustomed to the mask, he found that his sleepwalking stopped. He was also surprised to find that he was more alert during the day, though he had not noticed overt sleepiness prior to starting CPAP.

In part because he had a recent diagnosis of prediabetes too, a GLP-1 drug (Ozempic) was prescribed by his primary care physician. Not only did his blood sugar tests improve with subsequent weight loss, but his sleep apnea resolved as well, as shown by a follow-up sleep study, and his sleepwalking did not return when CPAP was discontinued. He and Ellen were delighted with these outcomes.

Any internal or external stimulus can set off an episode in a sleepwalker—a car horn outside, a noise in the bedroom, discomfort from a full bladder—if the sleeper happens to be in deep sleep at the time and if the stimulus occurs at just the right moment during deep sleep…and no one knows when that "right time" might be.

One of the most common triggers of sleepwalking activity is untreated sleep apnea (Chapter Four), as the multiple arousals from episodes of stopping breathing during sleep may produce that one special "strangulation event" that occurs at just the right time in deep sleep to promote an arousal that triggers sleepwalking. For this reason, all sleepwalkers should be screened for possible sleep apnea.

Sleep deprivation is also considered a trigger for sleepwalking, as sleep deprivation increases deep sleep the following night. Both excessive alcohol and caffeine have been implicated as causing sleepwalking, but both of these associations are considered controversial. Some researchers feel strongly that alcohol prior to sleep may increase sleepwalking, and others disagree. The same is true of caffeine intake. What is not controversial are the sleepwalking behaviors associated with some hypnotics, particularly Ambien. This is thought to be a form of drug-induced sleepwalking; what's more unusual about this is its common occurrence in those with no previous history of sleepwalking (see page 220).

After waking from a sleepwalking event, the sleeper usually has poor memory of the event. Occasionally the person can remember vague aspects of their motivation while asleep and may be able to describe in general terms what they were trying to accomplish; what they were searching for.

The range of things sleepwalkers do once they leave the bed can be fascinating. *Searching behaviors* are common. Vague wanderings are common, with no apparent goal, or the sleeper may wake another person and ask a nonsensical question. They might move furniture or pull a couch apart and then away from a wall trying to "find the baby" or something else. They might pull out drawers or open doors and closets searching for something. Urinating in a corner of the room or in a wastepaper basket is not uncommon, raising the question of whether a full bladder may have been the trigger to sleepwalk and the search for a place to relieve the pressure.

Scarier things, like opening a window or running down flights of stairs can occur, suggesting *escape behaviors,* and raising fears of injury. The comedian Mike Birbiglia, noted above, describes jumping out of a second-floor window while asleep and waking up on impact, not sure at first where he was or how he got there. Handling weapons like knives or guns is even more concerning. Sleepwalkers have been known to drive cars while asleep. They may arrive at their planned destination but their driving may not be perfect, perhaps missing stop signs and traffic lights. Worrisome.

Rochelle, 34, began sleepwalking in her 20s. Her husband Rick found her behavior amusing when they were first married, but later when he found that she had taken knives out of a kitchen drawer the previous night, he began to worry. When the noise of her unlocking and opening a second-floor door to a balcony woke him one night, he asked for a sleep medicine referral. Two days before her appointment, Rick found a burner on the stove burning when he went downstairs to the kitchen one morning; no one had used the kitchen at dinner time the evening before. Rochelle had no memory of any of these events.

Dr. Smith, the sleep physician, was concerned about the possible harms from all these dangerous sleepwalking behaviors. He excluded sleep apnea with a home study. His first recommendation, a side rail for her side of the bed, failed when she climbed over it when sleepwalking. Neither she nor Rick tolerated sleeping with a piece of string linking their wrists—a ploy to wake him if she left the bed—as they both became tangled in the string. Although Rochelle was not happy about it, Dr Smith then suggested she sleep in a zippered sleeping bag each night. Surprisingly, she tolerated this well and had no more dangerous behavior. Her sleepwalking attempts lessened as she aged and by her mid-40s she no longer had this problem.

Violent behaviors can also occur during sleepwalking, though rarely. When startled, a sleepwalker may lash out and hurt themselves or others, so trying to wake the sleepwalker (with shaking or yelling "wake up!" for example) may not be a good idea. Gently leading the sleepwalker back to bed is considered the safest approach; it's likely they will return to sleep quickly and not remember the incident in the morning.

Though rare, there are individual accounts in the medical literature of severe violence and even murder by sleepwalkers. In some cases the victim was known to the sleeper, but in others, the victim was a stranger. The legal defense of such activity, the ability of the defendant's attorney in persuading the jury that the sleeper was indeed asleep and therefore not responsible for their behavior, is key to preventing a guilty verdict and potential jail time.

Whenever a person accused of a crime claims that they were sleepwalking at the time, the onus falls on the defense to prove that the person was indeed asleep during the purported crime and therefore not responsible for their behavior. This can be difficult. In such situations, documenting a history and even a family history of previous sleepwalking may help, and the case for sleepwalking can be strengthened if witnessed sleepwalking can be induced in a sleep laboratory for forensic purposes, to be used by the defense in court. We will look at these techniques below.

At the end of the day, however, it is not possible to prove beyond doubt that a person was asleep at a particular point in the past; legally, the defense must persuade a judge and jury that the preponderance of the evidence suggests that the person was asleep when involved in bad behavior.

A classic way to induce sleepwalking for forensic purposes is to keep the person awake in the sleep laboratory for a period—say, 25 hours—of monitored sleep deprivation (to promote more deep sleep, more opportunity for sleepwalking), then perform a full sleep study with video monitoring.

When the technician detects deep sleep (by slow-wave activity on EEG), a brief stimulus, such as a short tone sent through headphones, is given to stimulate arousal. With luck (it doesn't always happen), an episode of sleepwalking may be induced right there in the lab, confirming the diagnosis and documenting it legally, with out-of-bed movements seen on video while simultaneous EEG recordings still show sleep.

These efforts are more useful in legal than in medical situations, as sleepwalking as a medical diagnosis is usually straightforward, acceptable as a diagnosis by descriptions by the sleeper and particularly from bedpartners, and doesn't require the effort and expense of the lab to confirm it. Having to prove it legally can be much more challenging.

Sleep violence is one variant of sleepwalking, obviously a serious one. Coverage in the media is not uncommon when these are uncovered, making these events notorious in the public mind.

One of the most famous cases of sleep violence[81] occurred in 1987 when 23-year-old Kenneth Parks drove 13 miles across Toronto, Canada, purportedly while asleep, and stabbed his mother-in-law to death. He was charged with first degree murder. He had turned himself in when he awoke after the event with blood on his lacerated hands, saying to the police "I think I have killed some people…" but he did not know who was involved until later when the event was described to him.

The defense relied on his personal and family history of sleepwalking, his amnesia for the event and his grief over the loss of his mother-in-law (with whom he was actually close), as well as his history of marked sleep deprivation prior to the event. His only other medical disorder was depression. Sleep experts testified on his behalf that the bulk of the evidence suggested that he was sleepwalking during the event, and therefore not legally responsible for his behavior. He was acquitted by a jury.

Cases of sleep violence are not common. A body of case law has grown in developed countries over the last few decades. A strong defense case presented to a receptive jury has in some cases, like that of Kenneth Parks, resulted in acquittal; in other cases, the jury has remained unconvinced that the defendant was unmotivated and, more importantly, even asleep during the commission of the crime, and has voted for conviction.

Remember the case I described at the very beginning of the book? It described another form of non-REM parasomnia, which has been called *sleep-sex*. Let's look at that case again:

In my role as a sleep specialist, I was occasionally asked to review legal cases in my field. This case became one of the most disappointing of all I reviewed.

In 2014, a 29-year-old man with a long history of sleepwalking and a family history of sleepwalking entered the bedroom and then the bed of an unrelated female at a house party, and had sex with her. She stated that she initially thought he was someone else and did not consider this rape until she recognized him after the event. He made no attempt to flee afterwards and seemed to have no recollection of the event when questioned. He was charged with felony rape.

At trial, where I testified as an expert witness, the jury and judge appeared receptive to my attempts to educate them about sleep and sleepwalking. Towards the end of the trial, the jury expressed wishes to find the defendant guilty of a misdemeanor, implying he should have known he might have sleepwalked at this house party—as he had sleepwalked at other times in this setting, and had a history of "sleep-sex" with his wife. The judge denied the jury's request, leaving them no recourse but to find him guilty of felony rape. The judge sentenced him to life imprisonment without chance of parole. Appeals were unsuccessful.*

I have been haunted by the thought of this innocent man languishing in prison for all these years. He remains in prison to this day.

Sleep-sex is categorized as a form of confusional arousal, perhaps a loose rule as some sleep-sex occurs after the sleeper has left the bed. As you might expect, sleep-sex encompasses all forms of sexual behavior, alone or with a partner, that occurs when the sleeper/performer is in deep sleep, including masturbation, sex-like "thrusting," touching or kissing or more serious sexual activity with a bedpartner, including penetration. This kind of behavior during deep sleep fits with our concept of emotion- or appetite-driven behavior, like the searching and escaping behavior in sleepwalking, and sleep violence and appetite-related sleep-eating.

Sleep-sex carries much more societal import than other parasomnias, with the possible exception of sleep-violence; since the sleep-sex partner may be seemingly randomly chosen, perhaps not someone acquainted

---

* She testified that they had had sleep-sex many times when she could tell he was asleep, and that his behavior and language during these events were markedly different from when they had sex when he was awake.

with the sexual actor, huge legal complications are not unusual, and the ultimate legal results may be very serious.

We can posit that sexual activity alone while asleep can be called harmless or victimless, though witnessing it while not understanding it may be distressing for others, particularly, perhaps, for children. Society does not condone the overt expression of sexual activity in the presence of adults without consent, or in the presence of minors. Actual sexual behavior with another during sleep may result in charges of sexual abuse or felony rape.

This highlights the most fundamental questions of what sleepwalking and its variants are, how they relate to the motivations and agency of the sleepwalker, and whether any level of culpability can be assigned to the sleepwalker, whatever the behavior. As in the sleep violence described earlier, prosecutors, defense counselors, judges, and juries may require extensive education in the subtleties of parasomnias, but even in the best of hands, the results may not be happy ones.

In criminal law, conviction of a crime generally requires both *mens rea* (a guilty mind) and *actus reus* (a criminal act). If I have a guilty mind about something (for example, I think about robbing a store) but no criminal act (I don't make any moves to rob the store, including conspiring with others to do so) then I cannot be convicted of a crime, as no crime has occurred. If I see my wife's lover on the sidewalk and decide to kill him, I clearly have a guilty mind. If I proceed to run him down with my car—clearly a criminal act—I can be convicted of a crime; I have satisfied both requirements.

But let's say I'm driving down the street and suddenly run up on the curb with my car and kill a stranger. This is potentially a criminal act; if I say it was accidental, I may still be held for negligent manslaughter. But now let's say that during the investigation after the accident, I am found to have a brain tumor that causes seizures, and that witnesses of the accident described me having seizure activity just after impact. My defense attorney will likely point out that I did not know the victim, and therefore had no motivation for harming him, and that I was having a seizure and therefore unconscious during the accident.

I did not have agency (the ability to decide to commit a crime and then act on it). I did not have a guilty mind and therefore did not commit a crime: it was an accident.

Now let's tweak this example another way. Let's say that I had been diagnosed with a brain tumor with seizures three weeks before the accident and was on anti-seizure medication. My neurologist had told me I could not drive for the next three months. Nonetheless, I still do drive, however, and have the accident described above. Am I guilty of criminal homicide? I'm not a lawyer, but I suspect I will be found guilty of negligence, perhaps negligent homicide.

I can now be accused of having *mens rea*, a guilty mind, in that I drove despite medical orders not to, despite knowing that I *might* cause an accident if I have a seizure. Also, my driving up onto the curb and killing someone now may be construed as *actus reus*, a crime, a crime of negligence. I can now be held to account in court and may be convicted. Same tumor, same seizure, same accident, same death, but in one case I'm innocent, the other guilty.

Clearly, the devil is in the details.

Back to sleep-sex. If a man exposes himself sexually to a stranger, that is a potentially criminal act: it's called *indecent exposure.* But if the man can be shown to have been asleep at the time of the exposure, then an enlightened court, with the assistance of good defense attorneys and expert witnesses, may find that he did not have a guilty mind at the time of the act, as he was asleep or "unconscious" when he exposed himself, and did not have the self-control we expect of our citizens in public.

If this happens, he stands a good chance of acquittal. Bolstering this claim that he was sleepwalking at the time—asleep when he exhibited sleep-sex, or in other cases, sleep violence—would be evidence that he had been a sleepwalker all his life, that he had a strong family history of sleepwalking, that he was sleep-deprived prior to the event, and that the event happened in the first third of the night.

But we can tweak this example too, as we did in the seizure/driving case. If it comes out in court that the man had a history of previous arrests for indecent exposure, especially during the daytime when he was less likely to be sleepwalking, the jury may not be convinced, no matter how good the evidence now, that he did *not* have a guilty mind. He may be found guilty.

This then is the dilemma of an attorney in defending a person (usually, but not always a male) accused of a sexual crime whose defense depends on his likelihood of being a sleepwalker. With the medical expert's help, the attorney must educate the court, the judge as well as the jury, about normal human sleep and its variants called sleepwalking and sleep-sex. The court must understand that there is case law in the US, in England, and elsewhere, where defendants have been acquitted of crimes committed while asleep, once it became apparent that those defendants did not have a guilty mind at the time of their purported crime, as they were asleep.

Since it is impossible to prove definitively that a person was asleep at any given point in the past, one can only hope to prove to a court that the preponderance of the evidence suggests the overwhelming *likelihood* that the defendant was asleep, and therefore not responsible for a crime. These efforts are not always successful.

Another variant of non-REM parasomnias is sleep-related eating.

Rosalie was a 47-year-old high school math teacher who noticed a 10-pound weight gain over six months' time. She noticed foods and non-food items, some partially eaten, on her kitchen counter in the mornings, including cupcakes, cake, and other sweets, but also unthawed frozen pizza, cigarettes coated in ketchup, and dried dog food in a bowl with milk. On a few occasions she found a gas burner still burning on the stove when she came into the kitchen in the morning.

She saw a sleep specialist who noted her family history of sleepwalking and her own history of confusional arousals from childhood into her teenage years. He excluded other sleep disorders by history and a sleep study, and diagnosed sleep-related eating disorder. He found that she had taken Ambien nightly for the past year, and, when this was stopped, all evidence of nocturnal eating resolved.

Sleep-related eating[82] is a form of sleepwalking involving mainly eating at night, rarely remembered, sometimes involving toxic substances or dangerous behavior, as with the gas stove above. It can occur on its own or in relation to other sleep disorders, like restless legs syndrome and sleep apnea, and to medications, most notably Ambien (but some antidepressants or antipsychotic drugs can do this too.) Females are more commonly affected.

Harriet's husband Jerry noticed that she sometimes moved at night in bed and was impressed that her movements seemed similar from one night to the next. She would sit up in bed and move her arms in a jerky fashion from side to side as in a crude hula dance; after a few minutes, she would lie back down and return to sleep. She never remembered these events and did not respond to his voice or gentle touch while she was moving. The events occurred at all times of the night.

She saw Dr. Smith, the sleep physician, who noted the stereotypical character of her movements (they always seemed the same pattern). He ordered an in-laboratory sleep study but, instead of four EEG leads, he requested 12, creating a larger than usual electrical map of the brain. By sheer luck, in the lab she performed her "hula dance" in the middle of the night, arising from light (N2) sleep. The EEG showed classic seizure activity in one part of the brain. She was diagnosed with sleep seizures, and was treated with anti-seizure medications with resolution of her nighttime behavior.

Confusional arousals can be confused with **sleep seizures**. Sleep seizures are *not* considered parasomnias, more an "electrical storm" in the brain, a problem thought to be from a series of abnormal electrical impulses arising from one spot in the brain and spreading out from there. We think of parasomnias more as "mistakes" made by the brain in dealing with arousal stimuli, with incomplete transitions into lighter stages, but no "storm." About 20% of seizures occur only during sleep.

Seizures may be suspected if the bedpartner describes jerky movements as seen in common seizures, with arching of the back and neck and rapid short movements of the limbs, or if *stereotypical behavior* is present, as in the same pattern of arm movements in multiple episodes over many nights. Ultimately, a sleep study with particular attention to EEG measurements of brain waves may be the only way to prove nocturnal seizures.

How is sleepwalking in general treated?

Treatment varies from as little as reassurance and/or gentle guiding back to bed, to medication, to aggressive restriction from dangerous places and devices. The treating physician must assess possible contributing disorders, such as sleep apnea, as well as the potential for harm, and will question the sleepwalker and family about medications and about any sleep behavior handling knives, guns, scissors, or other dangerous objects, as well as any risky behavior involving windows, doors, upper stories, staircases, and, of course, vehicles.

Treatment may include banning all dangerous objects from the bedroom, locking doors or placing alarms on doors and windows, moving the bed to the ground floor, and even restricting sleep to a zipped sleeping bag. Ensuring adequate sleep, reviewing medications, and screening for sleep apnea are all important too. Medical treatment is successful in some patients with clonazepam (a benzo), melatonin, and some antidepressants. Hypnosis has also been used.

The sleepwalker and their family members can sometimes be reassured that the incidence of sleepwalking tends to diminish as the incidence of deep sleep drops, namely, at the end of adolescence for many, and by the age of 40 for many more. This is not guaranteed, of course, but there is hope.

Sleepwalking can be mild or disruptive, entertaining or even dangerous. Abnormal eating, violence and even sexual activity may occur. Sleep seizures must also be considered. Full evaluation by a sleep physician is critical, especially in excluding other problems that may induce sleepwalking…such as sleep apnea. Sleepwalking may resolve on its own in many, but not all, cases, as the amounts of associated deep sleep drop off normally with age.

REM parasomnias

There are three sleep problems that occur during REM sleep: nightmares, sleep paralysis, and REM sleep behavior disorder (RBD). Let's concentrate on RBD, and start by re-reading Scenario #4 from our introduction into sleep disorders (see page 125):

Leo, 64, a lawyer, and his wife, Miriam, 59, are seeing Dr. Mitchell for his nightmares.

Miriam: "Dr. Mitchell, I am so worried about Leo. Every week or so he has a nightmare and begins yelling in his sleep, sometimes even kicking and punching. I can't wake him even when I yell back. See this bruise on my cheek? He hit me! But I know he didn't mean it—he was so apologetic after! What can we do?"

Leo: "I feel terrible about this, Dr. Mitchell. I tell myself it won't happen again but then it does. I usually am dreaming I'm being attacked by a man or an animal, and I have to fight my way out. Next thing I know I wake up with her yelling at me and I'm on the floor. I just can't go on hurting Miriam like this."

Dr. Mitchell: "I am going to adjust your diet and take you off all alcohol. I want to make sure you're getting enough sleep and maybe a vacation from work would help. I am also going to refer you for marriage counseling in case there is some underlying tension between the two of you prompting this kind of behavior."

Remember that this was a competent physician in 1965, hampered by his (and the world's) lack of knowledge about what we now recognize as RBD. Let's fast-forward 60 years, and now we have a modern-day sleep physician interviewing Leo and Miriam in 2025; some of the questions and answers in the interview might include the following:

Dr. Sleep: "Miriam, I know these events must be very disturbing for you. What wakes you when Leo has one of these?"

Miriam: "Sometimes he wakes me by moaning loudly, maybe just jerking his arms and legs a little. At other times he yells really loudly and flails his arms and legs. He's very strong and has hit me and kicked me while I'm yelling at him to wake up. It takes a long time for him to wake up even when I'm shouting at him. But when he wakes he's so sorry he has hurt me."

Dr. Sleep: "Leo, what do you remember about these events?"

Leo: "I'm usually having a dream, at first not really a nightmare, but at some point something goes wrong. Suddenly I'm next to a large snake, or being attacked by a large dog, or by a threatening man I don't know. I try to yell but no sound comes out. I try to get away but my arms and legs don't move well, as if I'm in jelly or mud. I try to kick the snake or the dog or the man but keep missing with my foot. I swing but my punches miss.

"Then I start hearing Miriam's voice way off, yelling at me to wake up—but I can't; it's too hard. When I finally wake I realize it has happened again—the bed is torn up and Miriam is standing over me and I feel terrible, knowing I've scared her and maybe hurt her. At times I've thrown myself out of bed and hit my face on my bedside table. Once I even got short of breath and found myself on the floor next to the bed with my head bent down on my chest in a weird way so my breath was cut off. I thought I was going to die."

Dr Sleep: "Miriam, what time of night do you think these dreams occur? Late at night, or early in the morning? Have you ever looked at the clock after one of these episodes?"

Miriam: "Funny you should ask! Some mornings I have to get up very early to go to work, so I look at the clock frequently to see how much more sleep I might get. I've looked at the clock a few times after the kicking and yelling calmed down. It's almost always late, after 4am or so."

In this example, our well-trained Dr. Sleep will have no problem making a preliminary diagnosis of RBD for Leo. Dr. Mitchell, as we have seen, would have had no chance of making an accurate diagnosis in 1965, as this disorder was neither described nor understood then. (That said, there is no reason to think that RBD was not affecting lots of patients then too. But none of them had any hope of help with it.)

This is an unusual but not rare disease: it affects less than 1% of patients over 60, and is more common in males (only 20% are female). It occasionally affects people as young as 43.* That said, many non-sleep physicians have never heard of it, even today. The difference for the RBD patient seeking a diagnosis for their dramatic problems in 2025 is that the average primary care physician now has connections with sleep physicians, and will refer someone this distressed even if they are not sure what the actual problem is.

There are basic elements of RBD that make sense once one recalls the normal physiology of REM sleep; other parts of the illness remain mysterious despite years of modern research.

Recall that an important feature of REM sleep is loss of muscle tone: it's *normal* to be almost completely paralyzed during REM sleep, a phenomenon that is thought to prevent us from acting out our dreams. The

---

* RBD can also occur in narcolepsy, which is also a disorder of REM-sleep regulation. This group is even younger, many in their teens and 20s. It is a milder problem then than when seen in older adults, and does not appear to have the same long-term consequences.

basic problem with RBD is the loss of that paralysis, the loss of what is called "atonia," or lack of muscle function. In RBD, the atonia is missing in REM, so the muscles still work and "dream-enactment behavior" occurs.

The clues to the diagnosis of RBD are nightmares usually in the last half or third of the night, when most REM occurs, with violent dreams and an unrestrained response to the dream with moaning, yelling, punching, and kicking; danger to the sleeper from falling from the bed and hitting furniture, and to the bedpartner from punching and kicking.

The diagnosis is strengthened by the finding of *REM sleep without atonia* (RSWA) on sleep studies. This means finding active electrical activity in the muscle channels (like the chin or leg muscles) during REM, rather than the flatlining on those channels that one would expect—meaning that muscle *tone* is present in REM, when it shouldn't be. Like sleepwalking, RBD occurs on random nights and the odds of seeing an actual episode while the patient is in the lab for a sleep study are small. We have to settle for looking for RSWA during a study to try to confirm our suspicion of this diagnosis, but may never see it.

Many patients, though, have stories so persuasive of RBD that sleep studies are not considered necessary for diagnosis. And there are patients with RSWA during sleep studies who do not have classical RBD.[83] Some patients with PTSD (post-traumatic stress disorder), for example, and many patients on antidepressants, can show RSWA on sleep studies. There is a theory that antidepressants may "unmask" RBD, given that RBD in patients on antidepressants seems to occur at an earlier age than in those not taking them.

Like sleepwalking, RBD may require preventative methods to prevent injury. Cushions placed around the sleeper to prevent collisions with furniture and falls to the floor may be necessary, as well as full-length cushions or pillows between the patient and bedpartner, to prevent bedpartner injury.

Lots of drugs have been tried to prevent these spells or lessen their frequency, but the two that seem to offer the most benefit are clonazepam and melatonin. Both may decrease frequency of events and the likelihood of injury. Melatonin may be more effective than clonazepam, and because clonazepam is a benzodiazepine, with all the problems that drugs in this class can cause (see page 211), many sleep physicians favor melatonin. Doses in the 3–15mg range are useful.

Now we come to the big elephant in the living room of all patients with known RBD: *there is a connection between RBD and dementia. RBD progresses to dementia in many patients after many years.*

When I first became aware of this connection from research literature perhaps 20 years ago, it was thought that perhaps 20% of patients with known RBD would go on to display dementia within nine to 12 years after diagnosis. Over the years since, the estimate has increased, to 30, then 50, and most recently 90%.

In other words, almost all patients with RBD may eventually, over a period of a decade or more after diagnosis, progress to dementia—which is terrible news. It's one thing to take a medicine nightly to prevent nightmares and violent behavior for an uncommon disease like RBD, and quite another to accept a future with a serious, family-destroying diagnosis like dementia that has no current treatment at all.

The dementias involved are not Alzheimer's; instead, they vary between rarer forms of dementia such as Lewy Body dementia, multiple system atrophy, and Parkinson's disease with dementia. It is now believed that RBD itself is a *prodrome*—like an early warning sign—of these forms of neurodegeneration, with the widespread nervous system damage that these illnesses entail. Still, not all patients with RBD do progress.

In the early years, when it appeared that only a minority of RBD patients might progress to dementia, many physicians did not feel it appropriate to alert RBD patients to this possibility. Why burden someone with the constant threat that they might develop a terrible, progressive, untreatable disease if the odds of getting it were low and the choices for stopping that development were *zero*? Who would choose to live with that knowledge? If dementia did emerge in an individual patient, then dementia-care—which is supportive only—could begin; if not, then the patient has been spared years of worry.

But that was when the odds were thought to be in the 20% range. Now that it appears that the majority of RBD patients are at risk, our attitude has changed. Discussions with patients and their families about the likelihood of future dementia are considered standard. These are not easy discussions: while there is treatment for RBD itself, as we have seen, there is still no standard method to prevent or treat dementia at this point.

But there is hope. As more is known about RBD and its progression, more can be done to prevent it. The North American Prodromal Synucleinopathy* (NAPS)[84] consortium is a collaboration of nine universities in the USA and Canada,[85] whose goals are to enroll and evaluate as many RBD patients as possible, to look for biomarkers of the different dementias, and to promote further research on prevention and treatment.

The ultimate goal is to develop *cytoprotection:* treatment that protects nerve cells, that prevents the degeneration of those cells that results in dementia, some approach that can be initiated as soon as RBD is diagnosed and the threat of future dementia anticipated. As of this writing, 2026, only one candidate for cytoprotection has been suggested: melatonin.[86] Animal studies have suggested that melatonin may offer a cytoprotective effect to prevent synucleinopathy progression. When equivalent doses for animals are calculated for humans, doses in the 40–100mg range are recommended, much higher than melatonin doses used for any other disorders. No research in human subjects with doses this high has been reported as yet.

Melatonin has strong antioxidant and other qualities that seem to inhibit cell death, which is the essence of cytoprotection. If indeed melatonin can prevent the downstream emergence of dementia, that will be a truly wonderful thing.

---

* *Synucleinopathy* means disease involving alpha-synuclein, an abnormal protein that aggregates in nerve cells and causes progressive damage. The various dementias and Parkinson's disease fall into this category.

REM sleep behavior disorder (RBD) can be dangerous for the sleeper and for the bedpartner. It heralds an uncertain future, with the daunting health risks of Parkinson's disease and dementia emerging years later. Diagnosis and treatment may be life-changing for both. Anyone exhibiting violent behavior during sleep should be evaluated by a sleep physician. Progression to devastating diseases is not assured for all, and treatment to prevent that progression appears to be on the horizon.

AFTERWORD

Every day in my digital news feed I find articles about sleep and sleep disorders, frequently more than one article a day. Sleep is a common topic for television and radio commentary too. It is gratifying to conclude that sleep is much more in the minds of health-conscious people now than, say, 40 years ago; good sleep is seen as an important activity promoting good physical and mental health, not just an inconvenient, time-wasting behavior to be minimized and avoided as much as possible. The military and the transportation industry now emphasize the value of sleep as never before.

As this book hopes to illustrate, what we have learned from research about sleep in the last 75 years is remarkable, and has the potential for changing all of our lives for the better. We now have the chance of sleeping longer and better, and having better mood, judgment, cognition, health, and even athletic ability using the tools we have gained in understanding human sleep. We have learned to recognize a number of sleep disorders whose existence was not known or even suspected years ago, and most are coming under control with behavioral and/or medical treatment.

This, to me, is a modern miracle.

So where might we go from here? What might the future hold for sleep medicine?

Let's explore a sleep physician's wish-list for the future: my hopes and expectations for where research may go for some of the bigger sleep problems. Some of these seem obvious next steps as new ideas for some sleep disorders; others are based on pure conjecture as to feasibility, but hopefully have some basis in reality.

Insomnia: This one is purely conjecture. The Holy Grail of sleep medications is a sleeping pill that induces natural sleep; "natural" in that all the sleep stages are present in age-appropriate amounts, that sleep time is normalized and that the induced sleep is as refreshing and rejuvenating as normal, unaided sleep. We would also demand of this perfect medicine that it achieve all of the more subtle benefits of normal sleep, namely enhanced memory functions (short- and long-term storage, discriminating forgetting, physical performance enhancement, and emotional regulation).

We require from that perfect pill that deep sleep in particular be maintained, or even increased, so that brain cleansing—glymphatic function—is preserved or even improved, hopefully decreasing risks of dementia. Finally, we want this medicine to have few side effects, to have no addiction potential, tolerance, or next-day impairment that might lead to accidents or cognitive problems.

We're not asking much! It is, after all, a wish.

Even more basic for insomnia, we wish that better understanding of the basic neuroscience of insomnia would lead to better understanding of the basic causes of insomnia, as well as leading to improved behavioral treatment. We have long known that those with chronic insomnia are *hyperaroused,* with higher cerebral metabolism, heart rates, and oxygen consumption. Why does this happen to some people and not others? What makes a person cross over from normal to hyperaroused, and how can that be reversed? Answers to these questions could make the development of the perfect sleeping pill unnecessary.

Obstructive sleep apnea: For OSA we could wish for a perfect medication too, one that might address the causes of the neural deficits seen in the soft palate and tongue base of OSA patients. Or better surgical procedures for sleep apneas, and better results. Or better CPAP machines, or, even better, more palatable (sorry!) ways to apply air pressure to the upper airway to keep it open at night, so the big problem of poor CPAP compliance is addressed. A form of clip-on hypoglossal nerve stimulator, avoiding surgery completely, would also be on my wish list.

A better explanation of the obesity epidemic of the last 35 years might lead to a return to normal of the average adult body mass index (BMI); this could eliminate two-thirds of all OSA cases that are related to obesity.

Lastly, we could wish that more understanding of the gender differences in OSA (men start as early as late teens/20s, women frequently not until after menopause) would result in better ways to avoid sleep apnea altogether.

On the diagnostic level, it's not unreasonable to wish that artificial intelligence will be applied to the analysis of sleep studies and eventually allow home studies that are as accurate as those done in the sleep laboratory, while becoming cheaper and easier to perform. There is still a large proportion of those with sleep apnea who remain undiagnosed.

Narcolepsy: Type 1 narcolepsy—the purest kind—is characterized by a deficit of the neurotransmitter, orexin. Getting replacement orexin into the brain is hard: giving it intravenously doesn't work, and putting it into the spinal canal is very difficult. One could wish for an oral version, that by some chemical manipulation could traverse the blood–brain barrier.

Better treatment, perhaps with drugs that fight sleepiness by providing alertness that more closely mimics that promoted by orexin itself, would be a step forward. Those with type 2 narcolepsy would likely benefit from this as well. Lastly, the genetic basis for narcolepsy is poorly understood. If stronger ties could be established, we would wish that genetic engineering could be applied to this lifelong illness that affects so many young people.

Idiopathic hypersomnia: This is sleepiness that mimics narcolepsy, but isn't. Our wish list includes better understanding (why does it happen? Why does it sometimes go away? What is the underlying problem?)

that would lead to more direct treatment, perhaps even with a goal of cure. Like narcolepsy, IHS would also benefit from better alertness-inducing medications, at least until our wished-for prevention or cure comes online.

REM sleep behavior disorder: Is this, as it appears to be, a predecessor of Parkinson's disease and dementia? We would wish that better understanding of the links between these problems would allow better treatment, with an eye toward stopping the disorder itself and particularly slowing or stopping the conversion to further neurodegeneration. This is neuroscience at its most basic, and has the potential for helping RBD patients and the larger group of Parkinson's patients. This extends our wish to helping millions, around the world.

As I write this, February 2026, there is a trend in Washington to cut off grants for all levels of medical research in this country in the name of budget control. For those of us in sleep medicine, that seems a terrible shame, given how far we've come in the last few decades. Almost all the progress discussed in this book stems from basic laboratory and clinical research, much of it funded by government grants in America. To lose this momentum would mean to lose any hope of wish fulfilment from our wish-list above, but more realistically would mean loss of that increase in knowledge and understanding that comes from day-to-day incremental research that is ongoing now.

Once that storm cloud of threats to research funding clears, I think the future of sleep medicine will be sunny. Research breakthroughs in sleep have a way of spilling over into benefits in non-sleep issues. For example, better understanding of RBD leads to better understanding of Parkinson's disease and the whole range of dementias; and better understanding of insomnia leads to better understanding of the neuroscience of anxiety and depression.

Since sleep occupies one-third of our normal existence, and the study of sleep entails exploration of the workings of the brain and the body, it follows that the knowledge of sleep gained may well benefit the other two-thirds of our lives: the "conscious" parts.

We have discussed a few of the thousands of great and small discoveries in sleep, both in the basic science and the clinical practice of sleep medicine, that have emerged over the last 75 years. Here's my main wish: that this will lead to better sleep for us all, with all the wonderful downstream effects that good sleep offers.

Sweet dreams.

NOTES

1. Ferber, R. *Solve Your Child's Sleep Problems*. Touchstone, 2006
2. Karp, H. *The Happiest Baby on the Block*. Bantam Books, 2015
3. Hobson JA. *Sleep*. Scientific American Library, 1989
4. Kleitman N. *Sleep and Wakefulness*. University of Chicago Press, 1963.
5. Rechtschaffen A, Kales A (eds): A manual of standardized terminology: techniques and scoring system for sleep stages of human subject. Los Angeles, UCLA Brain Information Service/Brain Research Institute, 1968.
6. Dement WC. *The Sleepwatchers*. Nychthemeron Press, 2nd ed., 1996.
7. Amini F, Moosavi SM, *et al.* Chronotype patterns associated with job satisfaction of shift working healthcare providers. *Chonobiol. Int.* 2021; 38: 526–533.
8. Borbely, A.A, Achermann, P. Concepts and models of sleep regulation: an overview. *J Sleep Res.* 1992; 1:63–79.
9. LazarusM, ChenJ-F, *et al.* Adenosine and sleep. *Handb Exp Pharmacol.* 2019; 253:359–381
10. Leenaars C, Savelyev S, et al. Intracerebral adenosine during sleep deprivation: a meta-analysis and new experimental data. *J Circadian Rhythms.* 2018: 16:11.
11. Dworak M, Diel P, *et al.* Intense exercise increases adenosine concentrations in rat brain: implications for a homeostatic sleep drive. *Neuroscience.* 2007; 150:789–795.
12. Greene R, Siegel, J. Sleep: A functional enigma. *Neuromolecular Med* 2004;5:59–68.
13. Tai Y, Obayashi K, *et al.* Hot-water bathing before bedtime and shorter sheep onset latency are accompanied by higher distal-proximal skin temperature gradient in older adults. *J Clin Sleep Med.* 2021; 17:1257–1266.
14. Ko Y, Lee J-Y. Effects of feet warming using bed socks on sleep quality and thermoregulatory responses in a cool environment. *J Physiol Anthropol.* 2018; 37:13.

15. Hirshkowitz M, Whiton K, *et al.* National Sleep Foundation's sleep time duration recommendations: methodology and results summary. *Sleep Health.* 2015; 1:40–43.

16. Seigel JM. "Evolution of Mammalian Sleep." In Kryger MH, Roth T, and Goldstein CA, *Principles and Practice of Sleep Medicine*, 7th ed., Elsevier, 2022:.93–105.

17. Helfrich-Forster C. Sleep in Insects. *Ann Rev Entomol.* 2018; 63:69–86

18. Ingiosi AM, Frank MG. Goodnight, astrocyte: waking up to astroglial mechanisms in sleep. FEBS J 2023. 290: 2553–2564.

19. Peever J, Fuller P. The biology of REM sleep. *Curr Biol.* 2017. 27: 1237–1248.

20. Wilson MA, McNaughton BL. Reactivation of hippocampal ensemble memories during sleep. *Science* 1984; 265: 676–682.

21. Niediek J and Bain J. Human single-unit recordings reveal a link between place-cells and episodic memory. *Front Syst Neurosci.* 2014; 8: 158–164

22. Li W, Ma L, *et al.* REM sleep selectively prunes and maintains new synapses in development and learning. *Nat Neurosci.* 2017; 30:427–437.

23. Yang G, Lai CS, *et al.* Sleep promotes branch-specific formation of dendritic spines after learning. *Science* 2014; 344: 173–178.

24. Walker M. *Why We Sleep.* Scribner, 2027. Chapter Five.

25. Xie L, et al. Sleep drives metabolite clearance from the adult brain. *Science* 2013; 342:373–377.

26. Moscoso, A, Grothe M. Time course of phosphorylated-tau 181 in blood across the Alzheimer's disease spectrum. *Brain.*2021: 144:325–339.

27. Himali J, Baril A-A, *et al.* Association between slow-wave sleep loss and incident dementia. *JAMA Neurol.* 2023 Oct 30. doi:10.1001/jamaneurol.2023.3889. Online ahead of print.

28. Shokri-Kojori E, Wang G-J, *et al.* Beta-amyloid accumulation in the human brain after one night of sleep deprivation. *PNAS* 2018; 115:4483–4488.

29. Hirshkowitz M, Whiton K, et al. National Sleep Foundation's sleep time duration recommendations: methodology and results summary. Sleep Health. 2015; 1:40–43.

30. Watson NF, Badr MS, *et al.* Recommended amount of sleep for a healthy adult: a joint consensus statement of the American Academy of Sleep Medicine and Sleep Research Society. *Sleep* 2015; 38:843–844.

31. Banks S, van Dongen H, *et al.* Neurobehavioral dynamics following chronic sleep restriction: dose-response effects of one night for recovery. *Sleep.* 2010; 33:1013–1026.

32. Pejovic S, Basta M, *et al.* Effects of recovery sleep after one work week of mild sleep restriction on interleukin-6 and cortisol secretion and daytime sleepiness and performance. *Am J Physiol Endocrinol Metab.* 2013; 305: 890–896.

33. Simpson N, Dilonbi M, *et al.* Repeating patterns of sleep restriction and recovery: do we get used to it? *Brain Behav Immun.* 2016. 58: 142–151.

34. Kim T, Jeong J-H, Hong S-C. The impact of sleep and circadian disturbance on hormones and metabolism. *Int.J. Endocrinol* 2015; 2015: Article ID 591729

35. Cappuccio FP, D'Elia L, *et al.* Quantity and quality of sleep and incidence of type 2 diabetes: a systematic review and meta-analysis. *Diabetes Care.* 2010; 33:414–420

36. Wu Y, Zhai L, Zhang D. Sleep duration and obesity among adults: a meta-analysis of prospective studies. *Sleep Med.* 2014; 15:1456–1462.

37. Zhu B, Shi C, *et al.* Effects of sleep restriction on metabolism-related parameters in healthy adults: a comprehensive review and meta-analysis of randomized controlled trials. *Sleep Med Rev.* 2019; 45: 18–30

38. Cuthbertson FM, Peirson SN, *et al:* Blue light-filtering intraocular lenses: review of potential benefits and side effects. *J Cataract Refract Surg.* 2009; 35:1281–1297.

39. American Academy of Ophthalmology, *Are Computer Glasses Worth It?* (updated October 4, 2021), https://www.aao.org/eye-health/tips-prevention/are-computer-glasses-worth-it.

40. Mednick S., Ehrman M. *Take A Nap! Change Your Life.* Workman Publishing; New York, NY, USA: 2006

41. Ekirch R. Segmented sleep in preindustrial societies. *Sleep* 2016. 39(3): 715–716

42. Yetish G, Kaplan H, *et al.* Natural sleep and its seasonal variation in three preindustrial societies. *Curr.Biol.*2015; 25: 2862–2868.

43. Thompson D. Can medieval sleeping habits fix America's insomnia? *The Atlantic,* January 27, 2022.

44. Freud S. *The Interpretation of Dreams.* Macmillan: 1913.

45. Tzioridou ST, Campillo-Ferer T, *et al.* The clinical neuroscience of lucid dreaming. *Neurosci Biobehav Rev.* 2025; 169: 106011.

46. Lerner B. A case that shook medicine. *Washington Post* Nov 28, 2006. Accessed online 01/03/2023.

47. Clinton J, Davis C, *et al.* Biochemical regulation of sleep and sleep biomarkers. *J Clin Sleep Med.* 2011; 15: S38–42.

48. Irwin M, Olmstead R, *et al.* Cognitive behavioral therapy and tai chi reverse cellular and genomic markers of inflammation in late life insomnia: a randomized controlled trial. *Biol Psychiatry.* 2015; 78: 721–729.

49. Martinez-Garcia M and Hernandez-Lemus E. Periodontal inflammation and systemic diseases: an overview. *Front. Physiol.* 2021; 12: 709438.

50. Frank MG, Heller HC. The function(s) of sleep. *Handb Exp Pharmacol.* 2019; 253: 3–34.

51. Young T, Peppard PE, and Gottlieb DJ. Epidemiology of obstructive sleep apnea: a population health perspective. *Am J Resp Crit Care Med* 2002; 165: 1217–1239.

52. Murray W. Johns, A new method for measuring daytime sleepiness: The Epworth Sleepiness Scale, *Sleep* 1991 14(6): 540–545.

53. Sullivan, C. Past, present, and future of CPAP. From a speech given to the National Sleep Foundation during Sleep Awareness Week, 2009. Accessed online 10/7/2012.

54. Abuzaid, AS, Al Ashry HS, *et al.* Meta-analysis of cardiovascular outcomes with continuous positive airway pressure therapy in patients with obstructive sleep apnea. *Am J Cardiol.*2017; 120: 693–699.

55. Balk EM, Adam GP, *et al.* Longterm effects on clinical event, mental health, and related outcomes of CPAP for obstructive sleep apnea: a systematic review. *J Clin Sleep Med.* 2024; 20: 895–909.

56. Jaganathan N, Kwon Y, *et al.* The emerging role of pharmacology in obstructive sleep apnea. *J Otorhinolaryngol Hear Bal Med.* 2024; 5: https://doi.org/10.3390/ohbm5020012.

57. Alrubasy WA, Abuawwad MT, *et al.* Hypoglossal nerve stimulation for obstructive sleep apnea in adults: an updated systematic review and meta-analysis. *Resp Med* 2024; 234: 107826.

58. Pappu A, Singh M. Best perioperative practices in the management of obstructive sleep apnea undergoing ambulatory surgery. *Curr Opin Anesthesiol.* 2014. 37: 644–650.

59. Dement WC. *The Sleepwatchers.* Nychthemeron Press, 2nd Ed., 1996.

60. Sonka K, Fekereova E, *et al.* Idiopathic hypersomnia years after the diagnosis. *Sleep Res.* 2024; 33(2):e14011. doi: 10.1111/jsr.14011.

61. Rishi MA, Ahmed O, *et al.* Daylight saving time: an American Academy of Sleep Medicine position statement. *J Clin Sleep Med* 2020; 16: 1781–1784.

62. Czyz-Szypenbejl K, Medrzycka-Dabrowska W: The impact of night work on the sleep and health of medical staff—a review of the latest scientific reports. *J Clin Med* 2024. 13:4505.

63. Wheaton AG, Chapman DP, and Croft JB. School start times, sleep, behavioral, health, and academic outcomes: a review of the literature. *J Sch Health* 2016; 86:363–381.

64. Videnovic A, Cai A. Irregular sleep-wake rhythm disorder: from the pathophysiologic perspective to the treatment. *Handbook Clin Neur.* 2025; 206: 71–87.

65. Stedman's Medical Dictionary, 21st edition. Williams and Wilkins, Baltimore, MD. 1966.

66. Stedman's Medical Dictionary, 27th edition. Lippincott, Williams and Wilkins, Baltimore, MD. 1999.

67. Stedman's Medical Dictionary. Wolters Kluver Health, Inc. Baltimore, MD. 2023.

68. Hornyak M, Scholz H, *et al.* What treatment works best for restless legs syndrome? Meta-analyses of dopaminergic and non-dopaminergic medications. *Sleep Med Rev* 2014; 18:153–164.

69. The International Classification of Sleep Disorders, 2nd Ed. American Academy of Sleep Medicine. 2005: 183.

70. Ferri R, Lanza G, and Mogavero MP. Strengthening the link between periodic limb movements during sleep and cerebral small vessel disease. *Sleep*, https://doi.org/10.1093/sleep/zsaf027. In press.

71. Woznica A, Carney C, *et al.* The insomnia and suicide link: toward an enhanced understanding of this relationship. *Sleep Med Rev.* 2015; Aug: 22:37–46.

72. Petersson H. The benzodiazepine withdrawal syndrome. *Addiction* 1994; 89:1455–1459.

73. Hou JH, Sun SL, *et al.* Relationships of hypnotics with incident dementia and Alzheimer's disease: a longitudinal study and meta-analysis. *J Prev Alzheimers Dis.* 2024; 11:117–129.

74. Chen P-L, Lee W-J, *et al.* Risk of dementia in patients with insomnia and longterm use of hypnotics: a population-based retrospective cohort study. *PLOS One* 2012; 7:e49113.

75. Billioti de Gage S, Moride Y, *et al.* Benzodiazepine use and risk of Alzheimer's disease: case control study. *BMJ* 2014; 349: g5205.

76. Kripke DF. I petitioned the FDA to restrict hypnotics: here is why. *Sleep Medicine* 2016; 23: 119–120.

77. O'Connor, A. New York Attorney General targets supplements at major retailers. *New York Times*, February 3, 2015.

78. Grigg-Damberger, M. Is there a better way to wean chronic benzodiazepine receptor agonists use by substituting a DORA (and starting CBT-I)? *J Clin Sleep Med.* April 1, 2024 https://doi.org/10.5664/jcsm.11058

79. Seyffert M, Lagisetty P, *et al.* Internet delivered cognitive behavioral therapy to treat insomnia: a systematic review and meta-analysis. *PLoS One.* 2016; 11: e0149139.

80. Birbiglia, Mike. *Sleepwalk with Me, and Other Painfully True Stories.* Simon and Schuster, 2010.

81. Boughton R, Billings R, *et al.* Homicidal somnambulism: a case report. *Sleep* 1994; 17: 253–264.

82. Vasiliu O. Current evidence and future perspectives in the exploration of sleep-related eating disorder—a systematic literature review. *Front. Psychiatry* 2024; 15: 1383337.

83. Feemster JC, Steele TA, *et al.* Abnormal rapid eye movement sleep atonia control in chronic post-traumatic stress disorder. *Sleep* 2022; 45: 1–12.
84. http://naps-rbd.org
85. Oregon Health and Sciences University, Stanford University, University of California Los Angeles, Washington University St Louis, Emory University, Massachusetts General University, McGill University, University of Minnesota, Mayo Clinic Rochester.
86. Cardinale DP and Garay A: Melatonin as chronobiotic/cytoprotective agent in REM sleep behavior disorder. *Brain Sci.* 2023; 13: 797–816.

GLOSSARY

2-AG 2-arachidonoylglycerol

ADHD Attention-deficit hyperactivity disorder

AHI Apnea-hypopnea index

AI Artificial Intelligence

ASPS Advanced sleep phase syndrome

ASV Adaptive servo-ventilation

BMI Body mass index

CBTi Cognitive Behavioral Therapy for insomnia

CHF Congestive heart failure

CO$_2$ Carbon dioxide

CPAP Continuous positive airway pressure

CR Circadian rhythm

CRP C-reactive protein

CSA Central sleep apnea

CSF Cerebrospinal fluid

DA Dopaminergic

DIMS Disorders of initiating and maintaining sleep

DOES Disorders of excessive sleepiness

DORA Dual orexin receptor antagonist

DPG Distal-proximal gradient

DSPS Delayed sleep phase syndrome

eCB Endocannabinoid hormone group

ESS Epworth sleepiness scale

EEG Electroencephalogram

EMG Electromyogram

ENT Ear, nose, and throat

EOG Electro-oculogram

EST Eastern Standard Time

FDA Federal Drug Administration

fMRI Functional magnetic resonance imaging

GLP-1 Glucagon-like peptide type 1

HNS Hypoglossal nerve stimulation

HST Home sleep studies

IHS Idiopathic hypersomnia

ICU Intensive care unit

IL-1 Interleukin-1

IR Infrared

ISWRD Irregular sleep-wake rhythm disorder

MAD Mandibular advancement device

MSLT Multiple sleep latency test

N1 Non-REM sleep stage 1

N2 Non-REM sleep stage 2

N3 Non-REM sleep stage 3 (also called delta sleep, deep sleep, or slow wave sleep)

N4 Non-REM sleep stage 4 (an outdated term)

N24SWD Non-24 hour sleep-wake disorder

NAPS North American Prodomal Synucleinopathy Group

Non-REM Any sleep that is not in REM sleep

NREM see Non-REM above

NT1 Narcolepsy type 1

NT2 Narcolepsy type 2

NYC New York City

OSA Obstructive sleep apnea

PLM Periodic limb movements

PVT Psychomotor vigilance testing

R REM sleep, as in sleep stage R

RBD REM sleep behavior disorder

RDI Respiratory disturbance index

REM Rapid eye movement sleep

RERA Respiratory-effort related arousal

RLS Restless legs syndrome

RSWA REM sleep without atonia

SAD Seasonal affective disorder

SAT Scholastic aptitude test

TNF Tumor necrosis factor

UPPP Uvulopalatopharyngoplasty

UP3 Uvulopalatopharyngoplasty

USP United States Pharmacopeia

UV Ultraviolet

W Wake, as in sleep stage W

ACKNOWLEDGEMENTS

This book took three years to write. Simple statement, but the writing itself took place in fits and starts, as I suspect it is for all but the most disciplined writers. I based the book, as you know, on all I had learned in 50 years of practice and studying sleep—but then in the process of researching the book, I learned a lot more. And I think there will always be more to learn, in sleep as in everything else, which is part of what makes life worth living.

From the very beginning of this project I leaned on friends, colleagues, and family for support, suggestions and critique. The final concept of the book is radically different from its original idea, in no small part from the support and advice from my wife Monica, my daughter Caroline, her husband Charles, my son Walt and his wife Felicity, as well as from Stephen Kennedy, Jim Braude, Tom Harbin, and Walter Jospin. Thanks also to Linda Klaitz, Alan Neely, Robert Wright, Don Bliwise, Marian Celli, Sheri Katz, Mike Egan, Michael Roach, and Kay Ashwood for all their support and critique. Maureen Corrigan gave critical analysis only an accomplished academician in literature could provide. Stephanie Waddell in the medical library at Piedmont Hospital in Atlanta was invaluable and tireless in running down reference books and medical articles for me. Rodel Lachica in the Sleep Laboratory at Piedmont Hospital helped me with real-time graphics from patients. Megan Hatfield created graphic beauty from my rough descriptions of sleep histograms. Bonnie Daneker and Esther Levine provided invaluable assistance in understanding the publishing world.

Above all, this project would not have ever been pursued, much less finished, had it not been for the love, support, and encouragement from *The Monica*…my wife. She applied her professional editing skills to every word and punctuation mark in the book (with deadly effects on most of my beloved semi-colons), and applied her years of college essay editing skills to raise the writing above pedestrian level. When the slings and arrows of outrageous manuscript rejections found their target, she nursed my emotional wounds back to health. That she has been my wife for more than three decades is the stuff of dreams.

This book is lovingly dedicated to her.

ABOUT THE AUTHOR

Walter James has recently retired after 50 years in the practice of medicine. He studied Applied Mathematics at Georgia Tech, Medicine at Tulane, and did postgraduate training in internal medicine and pulmonary disease at UC San Francisco and UC San Diego. He is board-certified in internal medicine, critical care, pulmonary diseases, and sleep medicine.

He founded The Sleep Center at Piedmont Hospital in Atlanta, Georgia, in 1992, and practiced clinical sleep medicine for 30 years, overlapping the practice of internal medicine, pulmonary medicine, and critical care. For a number of years he was a lecturer in sleep medicine at the Atlanta School of Sleep Medicine.

He is married, the father of two and grandfather of one. He enjoys historical reading, graphite drawing, and playing squash, pickleball, padel, and golf. His talent at the piano makes a good argument for recorded music.

If you'd like to connect with Dr. James, please send an email to wsj28g@gmail.com. If you are interested in newer information in the science of sleep, please visit his website at dreamingofanswers.com.